Current Clinical Strategies

Medicine

2001 Edition

Paul D. Chan, MD
Executive Editor

Michael Safani, PharmD
Assistant Clinical Professor
School of Pharmacy
University of California, San Francisco

Peter J. Winkle, MD
Associate Editor

Current Clinical Strategies Publishing

www.ccspublishing.com

Digital Book and Updates

Purchasers of this book may download the digital book and updates at the Current Clinical Strategies Publishing Internet site:

www.ccspublishing.com/ccs.htm

Current Clinical Strategies Publishing
27071 Cabot Road
Laguna Hills, California 92653-7012
Phone: 800-331-8227 or 949-348-8404
Fax: 800-965-9420 or 949-348-8405
E-mail: info@ccspublishing.com
Internet: www.ccspublishing.com

Printed in USA ISBN 1881528-83-9

Contents

Medical Documentation

History and Physical Examination

Identifying Data: Patient's name; age, race, sex. List the patient's significant medical problems. Name of informant (patient, relative).

Chief Compliant: Reason given by patient for seeking medical care and the duration of the symptom.

History of Present Illness (HPI): Describe the course of the patient's illness, including when it began, character of the symptoms, location where the symptoms began; aggravating or alleviating factors; pertinent positives and negatives. Describe past illnesses or surgeries, and past diagnostic testing.

Past Medical History (PMH): Past diseases, surgeries, hospitalizations; medical problems; history of diabetes, hypertension, peptic ulcer disease, asthma, myocardial infarction, cancer. In children include birth history, prenatal history, immunizations, and type of feedings.

Medications:

Allergies: Penicillin, codeine?

Family History: Medical problems in family, including the patient's disorder. Asthma, coronary artery disease, heart failure, cancer, tuberculosis.

Social History: Alcohol, smoking, drug usage. Marital status, employment situation. Level of education.

Review of Systems (ROS):

General: Weight gain or loss, loss of appetite, fever, chills, fatigue, night sweats.

Skin: Rashes, skin discolorations.

Head: Headaches, dizziness, masses, seizures.

Eyes: Visual changes, eye pain.

Ears: Tinnitus, vertigo, hearing loss.

Nose: Nose bleeds, discharge, sinus diseases.

Mouth and Throat: Dental disease, hoarseness, throat pain.

Respiratory: Cough, shortness of breath, sputum (color).

Cardiovascular: Chest pain, orthopnea, paroxysmal nocturnal dyspnea; dyspnea on exertion, claudication, edema, valvular disease.

Gastrointestinal: Dysphagia, abdominal pain, nausea, vomiting, hematemesis, diarrhea, constipation, melena (black tarry stools), hematochezia (bright red blood per rectum).

Genitourinary: Dysuria, frequency, hesitancy, hematuria, discharge.

Gynecological: Gravida/para, abortions, last menstrual period (frequency, duration), age of menarche, menopause; dysmenorrhea, contraception, vaginal bleeding, breast masses.

Endocrine: Polyuria, polydipsia, skin or hair changes, heat intolerance.

Musculoskeletal: Joint pain or swelling, arthritis, myalgias.

Skin and Lymphatics: Easy bruising, lymphadenopathy.

Neuropsychiatric: Weakness, seizures, memory changes, depression.

Physical Examination

General appearance: Note whether the patient looks "ill," well, or malnourished.

Vital Signs: Temperature, heart rate, respirations, blood pressure.

Skin: Rashes, scars, moles, capillary refill (in seconds).

Lymph Nodes: Cervical, supraclavicular, axillary, inguinal nodes; size, tenderness.

Head: Bruising, masses. Check fontanels in pediatric patients.

Eyes: Pupils equal round and react to light and accommodation (PERRLA); extra ocular movements intact (EOMI), and visual fields. Funduscopy (papilledema, arteriovenous nicking, hemorrhages, exudates); scleral icterus, ptosis.

Ears: Acuity, tympanic membranes (dull, shiny, intact, injected, bulging).

Mouth and Throat: Mucus membrane color and moisture; oral lesions, dentition, pharynx, tonsils.

Neck: Jugular venous distention (JVD) at a 45 degree incline, thyromegaly, lymphadenopathy, masses, bruits, abdominojugular reflux.

Chest: Equal expansion, tactile fremitus, percussion, auscultation, rhonchi, crackles, rubs, breath sounds, egophony, whispered pectoriloquy.

Heart: Point of maximal impulse (PMI), thrills (palpable turbulence); regular rate and rhythm (RRR), first and second heart sounds (S1, S2); gallops (S3, S4), murmurs (grade 1-6), pulses (graded 0-2+).

Breast: Dimpling, tenderness, masses, nipple discharge; axillary masses.

Abdomen: Contour (flat, scaphoid, obese, distended); scars, bowel sounds, bruits, tenderness, masses, liver span by percussion; hepatomegaly, splenomegaly; guarding, rebound, percussion note (tympanic), costovertebral angle tenderness (CVAT), suprapubic tenderness.

Genitourinary: Inguinal masses, hernias, scrotum, testicles, varicoceles.

Pelvic Examination: Vaginal mucosa, cervical discharge, uterine size, masses, adnexal masses, ovaries.

Extremities: Joint swelling, range of motion, edema (grade 1-4+); cyanosis, clubbing, edema (CCE); pulses (radial, ulnar, femoral, popliteal, posterior tibial, dorsalis pedis; simultaneous palpation of radial and femoral pulses).

Rectal Examination: Sphincter tone, masses, fissures; test for occult blood, prostate (nodules, tenderness, size).

Neurological: Mental status and affect; gait, strength (graded 0-5); touch sensation, pressure, pain, position and vibration; deep tendon reflexes (biceps, triceps, patellar, ankle; graded 0-4+); Romberg test (ability to stand erect with arms outstretched and eyes closed).

Cranial Nerve Examination:

I: Smell

II: Vision and visual fields

III, IV, VI: Pupil responses to light, extraocular eye movements, ptosis

V: Facial sensation, ability to open jaw against resistance, corneal reflex.

VII: Close eyes tightly, smile, show teeth

VIII: Hears watch tic; Weber test (lateralization of sound when tuning fork is placed on top of head); Rinne test (air conduction last longer than bone conduction when tuning fork is placed on mastoid process)

IX, X: Palette moves in midline when patient says "ah," speech

XI: Shoulder shrug and turns head against resistance

XII: Stick out tongue in midline

Labs: Electrolytes (sodium, potassium, bicarbonate, chloride, BUN, creatinine), CBC (hemoglobin, hematocrit, WBC count, platelets, differential); x-rays, ECG, urine analysis (UA), liver function tests (LFTs).

Assessment (Impression): Assign a number to each problem and discuss separately. Discuss differential diagnosis and give reasons that support the working diagnosis; give reasons for excluding other diagnoses.

Plan: Describe therapeutic plan for each numbered problem, including testing, laboratory studies, medications, and antibiotics.

Progress Notes

Daily progress notes should summarize developments in a patient's hospital course, problems that remain active, plans to treat those problems, and arrangements for discharge. Progress notes should address every element of the problem list.

Progress Note

Date/time:

Subjective: Any problems and symptoms of the patient should be charted. Appetite, pain, headaches or insomnia may be included.

Objective:

General appearance.

Vitals, including highest temperature over past 24 hours. Fluid I/O (inputs and outputs), including oral, parenteral, urine, and stool volumes.

Physical exam, including chest and abdomen, with particular attention to active problems. Emphasize changes from previous physical exams.

Labs: Include new test results and circle abnormal values.

Current medications: List all medications and dosages.

Assessment and Plan: This section should be organized by problem. Writing a separate assessment and plan should be written for each problem.

Procedure Note

A procedure note should be written in the chart when a procedure is performed. Procedure notes are brief operative notes.

Procedure Note

Date and time:
Procedure:
Indications:
Patient Consent: Document that the indications and risks were explained to the patient and that the patient consented: "The patient understands the risks of the procedure and consents in writing."
Lab tests: Relevant labs, such as the INR and CBC
Anesthesia: Local with 2% lidocaine
Description of Procedure: Briefly describe the procedure, including sterile prep, anesthesia method, patient position, devices used, anatomic location of procedure, and outcome.
Complications and Estimated Blood Loss (EBL):
Disposition: Describe how the patient tolerated the procedure.
Specimens: Describe any specimens obtained and labs tests which were ordered.

Discharge Note

The discharge note should be written in the patient's chart prior to discharge.

Discharge Note

Date/time:
Diagnoses:
Treatment: Briefly describe therapy provided during hospitalization, including antibiotic therapy, surgery, and cardiovascular drugs.
Studies Performed: Electrocardiograms, CT scan.
Discharge medications:
Follow-up Arrangements:

Discharge Summary

Patient's Name and Medical Record Number:

Date of Admission:

Date of Discharge:

Admitting Diagnosis:

Discharge Diagnosis:

Attending or Ward Team Responsible for Patient:

Surgical Procedures, Diagnostic Tests, Invasive Procedures:

Brief History, Pertinent Physical Examination, and Laboratory Data: Describe the course of the patient's disease up until the time that the patient came to the hospital, including physical exam and laboratory data.

Hospital Course: Describe the course of the patient's illness while in the hospital, including evaluation, treatment, medications, and outcome of treatment.

Discharged Condition: Describe improvement or deterioration in the patient's condition, and describe present status of the patient.

Disposition: Describe the situation to which the patient will be discharged (home, nursing home), and indicate who will take care of patient.

Discharged Medications: List medications and instructions for patient on taking the medications.

Discharged Instructions and Follow-up Care: Date of return for follow-up care at clinic; diet, exercise.

Problem List: List all active and past problems.

Copies: Send copies to attending, clinic, consultants.

Prescription Writing

- Patient's name:
- Date:
- Drug name and preparation (eg, tablets size): Lasix 40 mg
- Quantity to dispense: #40
- Frequency of administration: Sig: 1 po qAM
- Refills: None
- Signature

Advanced Cardiac Life Support

EMERGENCY CARDIAC CARE

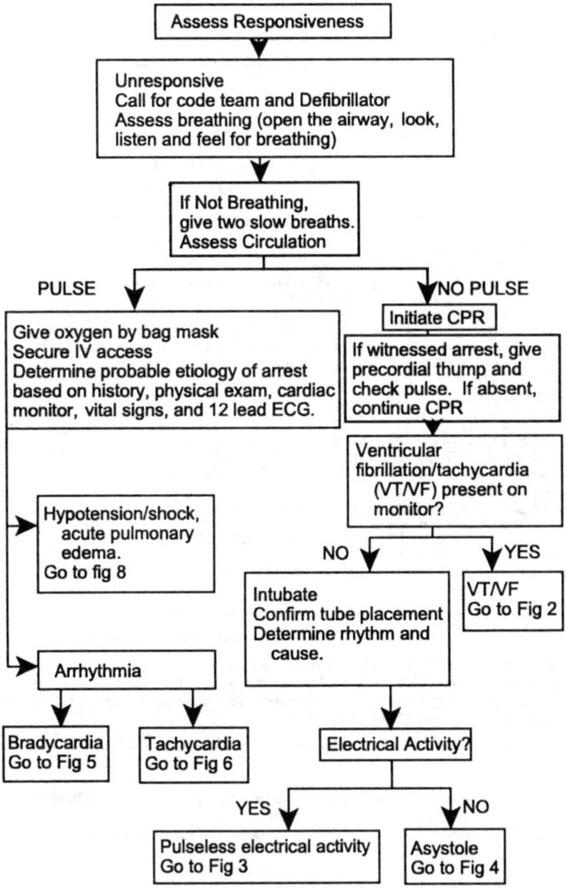

Fig 1 - Algorithm for Adult Emergency Cardiac Care

VENTRICULAR FIBRILLATION AND PULSELESS VENTRICULAR TACHYCARDIA

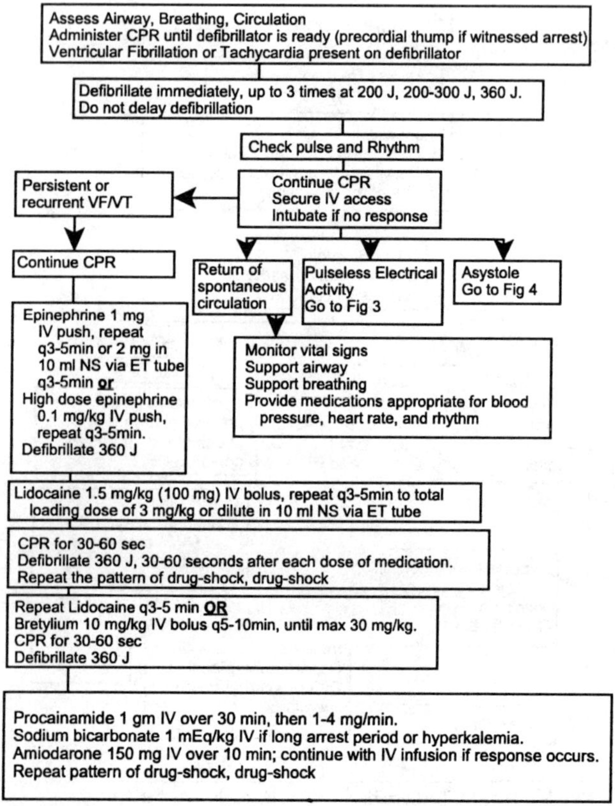

Note: Epinephrine, lidocaine, atropine may be given via endotracheal tube at 2-2.5 times the IV dose. Dilute in 10 cc of saline.
After each intravenous dose, give 20-30 mL bolus of IV fluid and elevate extremity.

Fig 2 - Ventricular Fibrillation and Pulseless Ventricular Tachycardia

PULSELESS ELECTRICAL ACTIVITY

Pulseless Electrical Activity Includes:
- Electromechanical dissociation (EMD)
- Pseudo-EMD
- Idioventricular rhythms
- Ventricular escape rhythms
- Bradyasystolic rhythms
- Postdefibrillation idioventricular rhythms

Initiate CPR, secure IV access, intubate, assess pulse.

↓

Treat Underlying Cause:
- Hypoxia (ventilate)
- Hypovolemia (infuse volume)
- Pericardial tamponade (performpericardiocentesis)
- Tension pneumothorax (perform needle decompression)
- Pulmonary embolism (thrombectomy, thrombolytics)
- Drug overdose with tricyclics, digoxin, beta, or calcium blockers
- Hyperkalemia or hypokalemia
- Acidosis (give bicarbonate)
- Myocardial infarction (thrombolytics)
- Hypothemia (active rewarming)

↓

Epinephrine 1.0 mg IV bolus q3-5 min, or high dose epinephrine 0.1 mg/kg IV push q3-5 min; may give via ET tube.
Continue CPR

↓

If bradycardia (<60 beats/min), give atroprine 1 mg IV, q3-5 min, up to total of 0.04 mg/kg
Consider bicarbonate, 1 mEq/kg IV (1-2 amp, 44 mEq/amp), if hyperkalemia or other indications.

Fig 3 - Pulseless Electrical Activity

ASYSTOLE

Continue CPR. Confirm asystole by repositioning paddles or by checking 2 leads. Intubate and secure IV access.

↓

Consider underlying cause, such as hypoxia, hyperkalemia, hypokalemia, acidosis, drug overdose, hypothermia. myocardial infarction.

↓

Consider transcutaneous pacing (TCP)

↓

Epinephrine 1.0 mg IV push, repeat every 3-5 min; may give by ET tube; high dose epinephrine 0.1 mg/kg IV push q5min (1:1000 sln).

↓

Atropine 1 mg IV, repeat q3-5min up to a total of 0.04 mg/kg; may give via ET tube.

↓

Consider bicarbonate 1 mEq/kg (1-2 amp) if hyperkalemia, acidosis, tricyclic overdose. Consider termination of efforts.

Fig 4 - Asystole

BRADYCARDIA

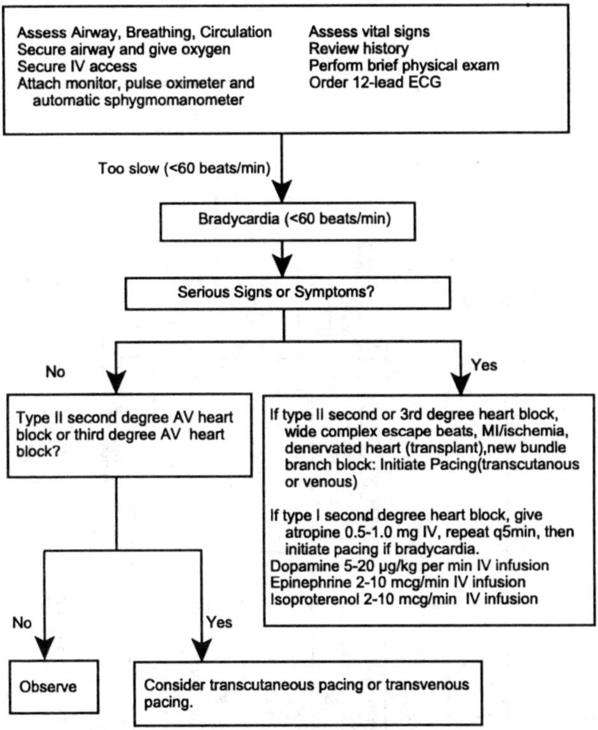

Fig 5 - Bradycardia (with patient not in cardiac arrest).

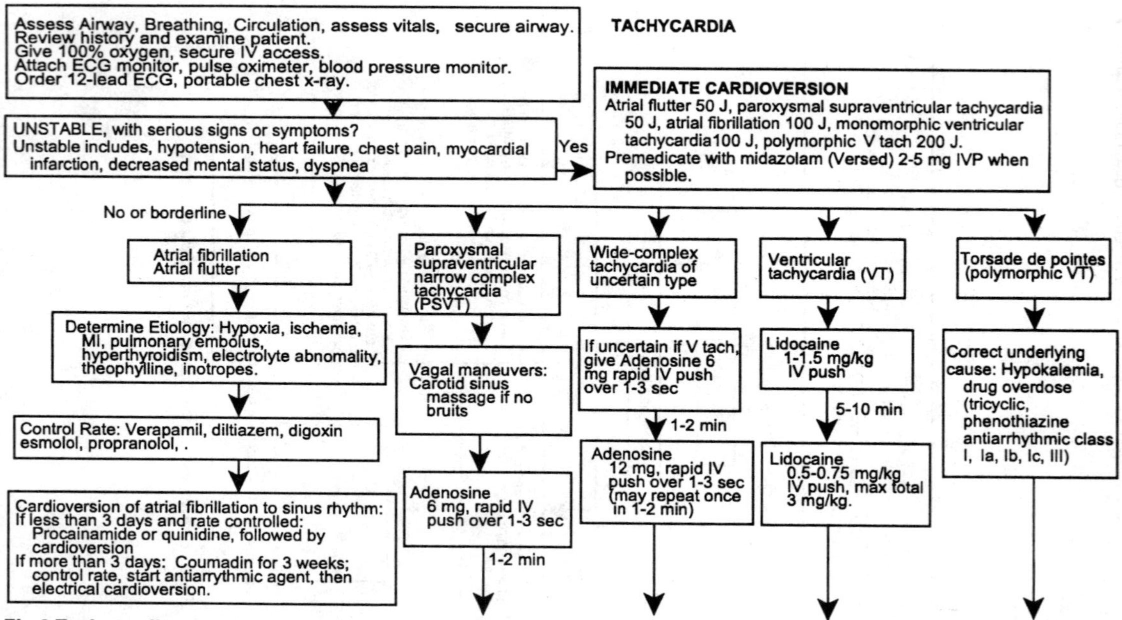

Fig 6 Tachycardia

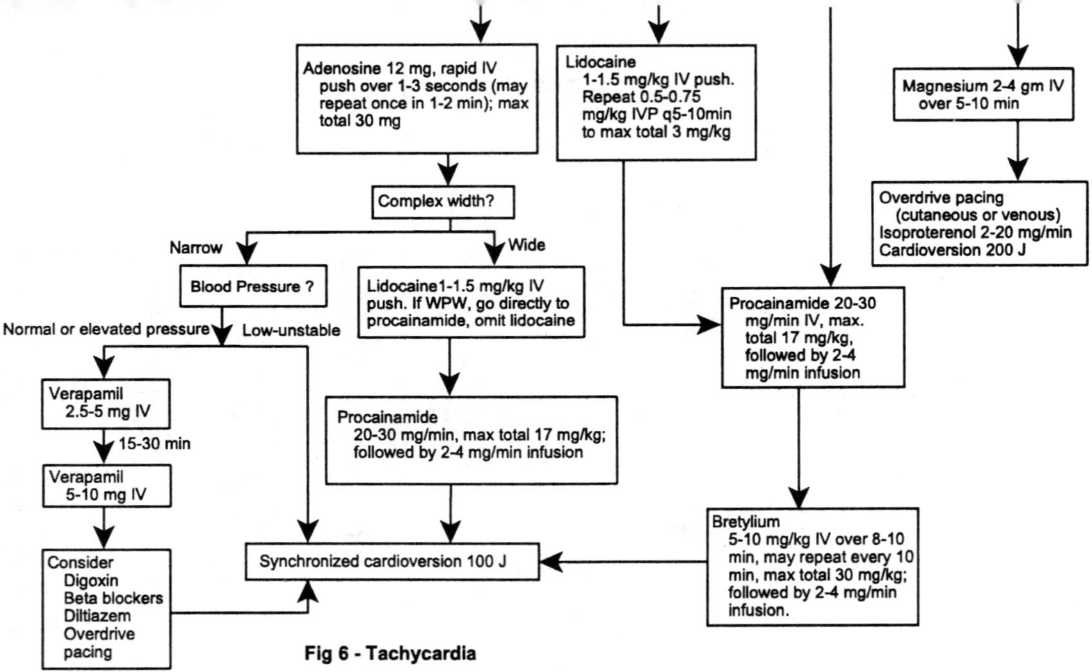

Fig 6 - Tachycardia

STABLE TACHYCARDIA

Stable tachycardia with serious signs and symptoms related to the tachycardia. Patient not in cardiac arrest.

↓

If ventricular rate is >150 beats/min, prepare for immediate cardioversion. **Treatment of Stable Patients is based on Arrhythmia Type:**

V-Tach: Lidocaine 1-1.5 mg/kg IVP, then 0.5-0.75 mg/kg q5-10min to max total 3 mg/kg. If no response, give procainamide 20-30 mg/min to max total 17 mg/kg, or bretylium 5-10 mg/kg over 8-10minutes, q10min to max total 30 mg/kg.

Paroxysmal Supraventricular Tachycardia: Carotid sinus pressure (if bruits absent), then adenosine 6 mg rapid IVP, followed by 12 mg rapid IVP x 2 doses to max total 30 mg. If no response, verapamil 2.5-5.0 mg IVP; may repeat dose with 5-10 mg IVP if adequate blood pressure; or Esmolol 500 mcg/kg IV over 1 min, then 50 mcg/kg/min IV infusion, and titrate up to 200 mcg/kg/min IV infusion.

Atrial Fibrillation/Flutter: Digoxin 0.5 mg IVP followed by 0.25 mg IVP q4h x 2-4 doses for rate control, then procainamide 20-30 mg/min IV to total max of 17 mg/kg, followed by 2-4 mg/min IV infusion.

↓

Check oxygen saturation, suction device, intubation equipment. Secure IV access

↓

Premedicate whenever possible with Midazolam (Versed) 2-5 mg IVP or sodium pentothal 2 mg/kg rapid IVP

↓

Synchronized cardioversion

Atrialflutter	50 J
PSVT	50 J
Atrial	100 J
Monomorphic V-tach	100 J
Polymorphic V tach	200 J

Fig 7 - Stable Tachycardia (not in cardiac arrest)

HYPOTENSION, SHOCK, AND ACUTE PULMONARY EDEMA

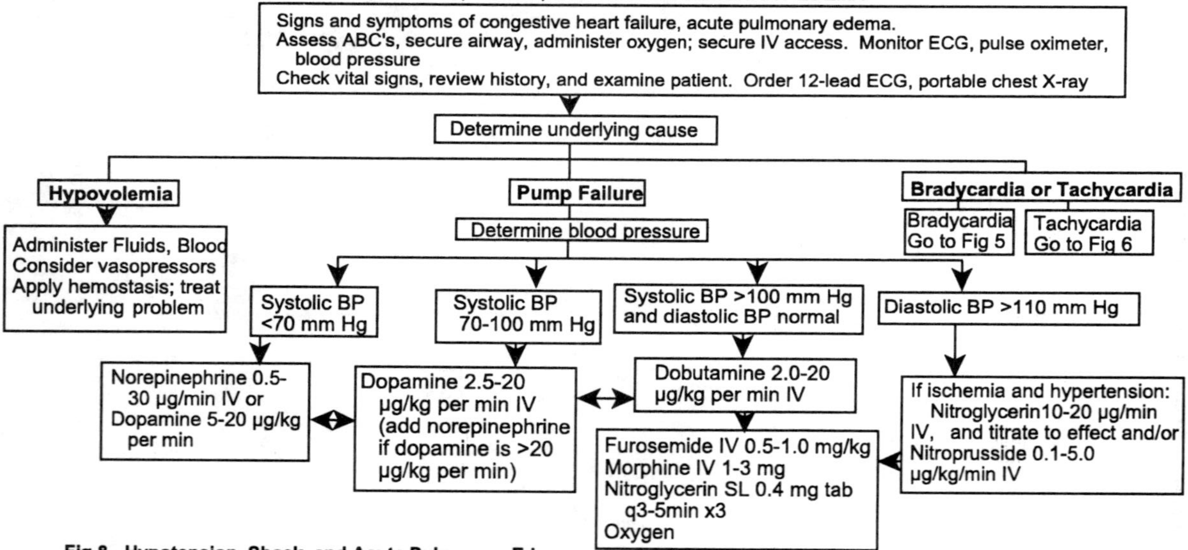

Fig 8 - Hypotension, Shock, and Acute Pulmonary Edema

Cardiovascular Disorders

Myocardial Infarction and Unstable Angina

1. **Admit to:** Coronary care unit
2. **Diagnosis:** Rule out myocardial infarction
3 **Condition:**
4. **Vital signs:** q1h. Call physician if pulse >90,<60; BP >150/90, <90/60; R>25, <12; T >38.5°C.
5. **Activity:** Bed rest with bedside commode.
7. **Nursing:** Guaiac stools. If patient has chest pain, obtain 12-lead ECG and call physician.
8. **Diet:** Cardiac diet, 1-2 gm sodium, low fat, low cholesterol diet. No caffeine or temperature extremes.
9. **IV Fluids:** D5W at TKO
10. **Special Medications:**
 -Oxygen 2-4 L/min by NC.
 -Aspirin 325 mg PO, chew and swallow, then 160 mg PO qd **OR**
 -Clopidogrel (Plavix) 300 mg PO x 1, then 75 mg PO qd (if allergic to aspirin).
 -Nitroglycerine infusion 15 mcg IV bolus, then 10 mcg/min infusion (50 mg in 250-500 mL D5W, 100-200 mcg/mL). Titrate to control symptoms in 5-10 mcg/min steps, up to 200-300 mcg/min; maintain systolic BP >90 **OR**
 -Nitroglycerine SL, 0.4 mg (0.15-0.6 mg) SL q5min until pain free (up to 3 tabs) **OR**
 -Nitroglycerin spray (0.4 mg/aerosol spray) 1-2 sprays under the tongue q 5min; MR x 2.
 -Heparin 75 U/kg IV push, then 15 U/kg/hr by continuous IV infusion.
 -aPTTq6h x 4, then qd. Repeat aPTT 6 hours after each heparin dosage change.

Glycoprotein II_b/III_a Blockers for Acute Coronary Syndromes:
 -**Eptifibatide (Integrilin)** 180mcg/kg IVP, then 2 mcg/kg/min for 72 hours.
 -**Tirofiban (Aggrastat)** 0.4 mcg/kg/min for 30 min, then 0.1 mcg/kg/min for 48-108 hours.

Glycoprotein IIb/IIIa blockers for Use With Angioplasty:
 -**Abciximab (ReoPro)** 0.25 mg/kg IVP, then 0.125 mcg/kg/min IV infusion for 12 hours.
 -**Eptifibatide (Integrilin)** 180 mcg/kg IVP, then 2 mcg/kg/min for 20-24 hours.

Thrombolytic Therapy

Absolute Contraindications to Thrombolytics: Active internal bleeding, history of hemorrhagic stroke, head trauma, pregnancy, surgery within 2 wk, recent non-compressible vascular puncture, uncontrolled hypertension (>180/110 mmHg).

Relative Contraindications to Thrombolytics: Absence of ST-segment elevation, severe hypertension, cerebrovascular disease, recent surgery (within 2 weeks), cardiopulmonary resuscitation.

A. Alteplase (tPA, recombinant tissue plasminogen activator, Activase):

1. 15 mg IV push over 2 min, followed by 0.75 mg/kg (max 50 mg) IV infusion over 30 min, followed by 0.5 mg/kg (max 35 mg) IV infusion over 60 min (max total dose 100 mg).
2. **Labs:** INR/PTT, CBC, fibrinogen.

B. Reteplase (Retavase):

1. 10 U IV push over 2 min; repeat second 10 U IV push after 30 min.
2. **Labs:** INR, aPTT, CBC, fibrinogen.

C. Streptokinase (Streptase):

1. 1.5 million IU in 100 mL NS IV over 60 min. Pretreat with diphenhydramine (Benadryl) 50 mg IV push **AND** Methylprednisolone (Soln-Medrol) 250 mg IV push.
2. Check fibrinogen level now and q6h for 24h until level >100 mg/dL.
3. No IM or arterial punctures, watch IV for bleeding.

Angiotensin Converting Enzyme Inhibitors:

-Captopril (Capoten) initial dose 6.25 mg PO; after 2 hours, increase to 12.5 mg; after 6-8 hours, increase to 25 mg, then increase to 50 mg bid on day 2 **OR**

-Lisinopril (Zestril, Prinivil) 5 mg PO x 1 dose, then 10 mg qd, then 10-20 mg bid.

-Enalapril (Vasotec) 2.5 mg PO x 1, then 5 mg qd. Increase dose to max dose of 10-20 mg bid.

Long-acting Nitrates:

-Nitroglycerin patch 0.2 mg/hr qd. Allow for nitrate-free period to prevent tachyphylaxis.

-Isosorbide dinitrate (Isordil) 10-60 mg PO tid [5,10,20, 30,40 mg] **OR**

-Isosorbide mononitrate (Imdur) 30-60 mg PO qd.

Beta-Blockers: Contraindicated in cardiogenic shock.

-Metoprolol (Lopressor) 5 mg IV q2-5min x 3 doses; then 25 mg PO q6h for 48h, then 100 mg PO q12h; keep HR <60/min, hold if systolic BP <100 mmHg **OR**

-Atenolol (Tenormin), 5 mg IV, repeated in 5 minutes, followed by 50-100 mg PO qd **OR**

-Esmolol hydrochloride (Brevibloc) 500 mcg/kg IV over 1 min, then 50 mcg/kg/min IV infusion, titrated to heart rate >60 bpm (max 300 mcg/kg/min).

11. Symptomatic Medications:

-Morphine sulfate 2-4 mg IV push prn chest pain.

-Acetaminophen (Tylenol) 325-650 mg PO q4-6h prn headache.

-Lorazepam (Ativan) 1-2 mg PO tid-qid prn anxiety

-Zolpidem (Ambien) 5-10 mg qhs prn insomnia.

-Docusate (Colace) 100 mg PO bid.

-Dimenhydrinate (Dramamine) 25-50 mg IV over 2-5 min q4-6h or 50 mg PO q4-6h prn nausea.

-Ranitidine (Zantac) 150 mg PO bid or 50 mg IV q8h.

12. Extras: ECG stat and in 12h and in AM, portable CXR. Cardiology consult.

13. **Labs:** SMA7 and 12, magnesium. Cardiac enzymes: CPK-MB, troponin T STAT and q6h for 24h. LDH and isoenzymes. CBC, INR/PTT, UA.

Congestive Heart Failure

1. **Admit to:**
2. **Diagnosis:** Congestive Heart Failure
3. **Condition:**
4. **Vital signs:** q1h. Call physician if P >120; BP >150/100 <80/60; T >38.5°C; R >25, <10.
5. **Activity:** Bed rest with bedside commode.
6. **Nursing:** Daily weights, measure inputs and outputs. Head-of-bed at 45 degrees, legs elevated.
7. **Diet:** 1-2 gm salt, cardiac diet.
8. **IV Fluids:** Heparin lock with flush q shift.
9. **Special Medications:**

-Oxygen 2-4 L/min by NC.

Diuretics:

-Furosemide 10-160 mg IV qd-bid or 20-80 mg PO qAM-bid [20,40,80 mg] **OR**

-Torsemide (Demadex) 10-40 mg IV or PO qd; max 200 mg/day [5, 10, 20, 100 mg] **OR**

-Bumetanide (Bumex) 0.5-1 mg IV q2-3h until response; then 0.5-1.0 mg IV q8-24h (max 10 mg/d); or 0.5-2.0 mg PO qAM.

-Metolazone (Zaroxolyn) 2.5-10 mg PO qd, max 20 mg/d; 30 min before loop diuretic [2.5,5,10 mg].

ACE Inhibitors:

-Quinapril (Accupril) 5-10 mg PO qd x 1 dose, then 20-80 mg PO qd in 1 to 2 divided doses [5,10,20,40 mg] **OR**

-Lisinopril (Zestril, Prinivil) 5-40 mg PO qd [5,10,20,40 mg] **OR**

-Benazepril (Lotensin) 10-40 mg PO qd, max 80 mg/d [5,10,20,40 mg] **OR**

-Fosinopril (Monopril) 10-40 mg PO qd, max 80 mg/d [10,20 mg] **OR**

-Ramipril (Altace) 2.5-10 mg PO qd, max 20 mg/d [1.25,2.5,5,10 mg].

-Captopril (Capoten) 6.25-50 mg PO q8h [12.5, 25,50,100 mg] **OR**

-Enalapril (Vasotec) 1.25-5 mg slow IV push q6h or 2.5-20 mg PO bid [5,10,20 mg] **OR**

-Moexipril (Univasc) 7.5 mg PO qd x 1 dose, then 7.5-15 mg PO qd-bid [7.5, 15 mg tabs] **OR**

-Trandolapril (Mavik) 1 mg qd x 1 dose, then 2-4 mg qd [1, 2, 4 mg tabs].

Angiotensin-II Receptor Blockers:

-Irbesartan (Avapro) 150 mg qd, max 300 mg qd [75, 150, 300 mg].

-Losartan (Cozaar) 25-50 mg bid [25, 50 mg].

-Valsartan (Diovan) 80 mg qd; max 320 mg qd [80, 160 mg].

-Candesartan (Atacand) 8-16 mg qd-bid [4, 8, 16, 32 mg].

-Telmisartan (Micardis) 40-80 mg qd [40, 80 mg].

Beta-blockers:

-Carvedilol (Coreg) 3.125 mg PO bid, then slowly increase the dose every 2 weeks to max 25 mg PO bid if <85 kg or 50 mg PO bid if > 85 kg. [tab 3.125, 6.25, 12.5, 25 mg] **OR**

-Metoprolol (Lopressor) 6.25 mg PO bid, then 12.5-50 mg PO bid [50, 100 mg].

-Bisoprolol (Zebeta) 2.5-10 mg qd; max 20 mg qd [5,10 mg].

Digoxin: (Lanoxin) 0.125-0.5 mg PO or IV qd [0.125,0.25, 0.5 mg].

Inotropic Agents:

-Dopamine (Intropin) 3-15 mcg/kg/min IV (400 mg in 250 cc D5W, 1600 mcg/mL), titrate to CO >4, CI >2; systolic >90 **OR**

-Dobutamine (Dobutrex) 2.5-10 mcg/kg/min IV, max of 14 mcg/kg/min (500 mg in 250 mL D5W, 2 mcg/mL) **AND/OR**

-Milrinone (Primacor) 50 mcg/kg IV over 10 min, followed by 0.375-0.75 mcg/kg/min IV infusion (40 mg in 200 mL NS, 0.2 mg/mL); arrhythmogenic; may cause hypotension

Potassium:

-KCL (Micro-K) 20-60 mEq PO qd.

10. Symptomatic Medications:

-Morphine sulfate 2-4 mg IV push prn dyspnea or anxiety.

-Heparin 5000 U SQ q12h.

-Docusate sodium 100-200 mg PO qhs.

-Ranitidine (Zantac)150 mg PO bid or 50 mg IV q8h.

11. Extras: CXR PA and LAT, ECG now and repeat if chest pain or palpitations.

12. Labs: SMA 7&12, CBC; cardiac enzymes: CPK-MB, troponin T STAT and q6h for 24h. Repeat SMA 7 in AM. UA.

Supraventricular Tachycardia

1. **Admit to:**
2. **Diagnosis:** PSVT
3. **Condition:**
4. **Vital signs:** q1h. Call physician if BP >160/90, <90/60; apical pulse >130, <50; R >25, <10; T >38.5°C
5. **Activity:** Bedrest with bedside commode.
6. **Nursing:**
7. **Diet:** Low fat, low cholesterol, no caffeine.
8. **IV Fluids:** D5W at TKO.
9. **Special Medications:**

Attempt vagal maneuvers (Valsalva maneuver and/or carotid sinus massage) before drug therapy.

Cardioversion (if unstable or refractory to drug therapy):

1. NPO for 6h, digoxin level must be less than 2.4 and potassium and magnesium must be normal.
2. Midazolam (Versed) 2-5 mg IV push.
3. If stable, cardiovert with synchronized 10-50 J, and increase by 50 J incre-

ments if necessary. If unstable, start with 75-100 J, then increase to 200 J and 360 J.

Pharmacologic Therapy of Supraventricular Tachycardia:

-Adenosine (Adenocard) 6 mg rapid IV over 1-2 sec, followed by saline flush, may repeat 12 mg IV after 2-3 min, up to max of 30 mg total **OR**

-Verapamil (Isoptin) 2.5-5 mg IV over 2-3min (may give calcium gluconate 1 gm IV over 3-6 min prior to verapamil); then 40-120 mg PO q8h [40, 80, 120 mg] or verapamil SR 120-240 mg PO qd [120, 180, 240 mg] **OR**

-Esmolol hydrochloride (Brevibloc) 500 mcg/kg IV over 1 min, then 50 mcg/kg/min IV infusion titrated to HR of <60 (max of 300 mcg/kg/min) **OR**

-Diltiazem (Cardizem) 0.25 mg/kg IV over 2-5 minutes **OR**

-Propranolol 1-5 mg (0.15 mg/kg) given IV in 1 mg aliquots; then propranolol-LA 60-320 mg PO qd [60, 80, 120, 160 mg] OR

-Digoxin 0.25 mg q4h as needed; up to 1.0-1.5 mg; then 0.125-0.25 mg PO qd.

10.Symptomatic Medications:

-Lorazepam (Ativan) 1-2 mg PO tid prn anxiety.

11.Extras: Portable CXR, ECG; repeat if chest pain. Cardiology consult.

12.Labs: CBC, SMA 7&12, Mg, thyroid panel. UA.

Ventricular Arrhythmias

1. **Ventricular Fibrillation and Tachycardia:**

   -**If unstable (see ACLS protocol):** Defibrillate with unsynchronized 200 J, then 300 J.

   -Oxygen 100% by mask.

   -Lidocaine (Xylocaine) loading dose 75-100 mg IV, then 2-4 mg/min IV **OR**

   -Bretylium (Bretylol) loading dose 5-10 mg/kg over 5-10 min, then 1-4 mg/min IV infusion.

   -Amiodarone (Cordarone) 150 mg in 100 mL of D5W, IV infusion over 10 min, then 900 mg in 500 mL of D5W, at 1 mg/min for 6 hrs, then at 0.5 mg/min thereafter.

   -**Also see "other antiarrhythmics" below.**

2. **Torsades De Pointes Ventricular Tachycardia:**

   -Correct underlying cause and consider discontinuing quinidine, procainamide, disopyramide, moricizine, lidocaine, amiodarone, sotalol, cisapride, Ibutilide, phenothiazine, haloperidol, tricyclic and tetracyclic antidepressants, ketoconazole, itraconazole, bepridil, hypokalemia, and hypomagnesemia.

   -Magnesium sulfate 1-4 gm in IV bolus over 5-15 min or infuse 3-20 mg/min for 7-48h until QT interval <440 msec.

   -Isoproterenol (Isuprel), 2-20 mcg/min (2 mg in 500 mL D5W, 4 mcg/mL).

   -Consider ventricular pacing and/or cardioversion.

3. Other Antiarrhythmics:

Class I:

-Moricizine (Ethmozine) 200-300 mg PO q8h, max 900 mg/d [200, 250, 300 mg].

Class Ia:

-Quinidine gluconate (Quinaglute) 324-648 mg PO q8-12h [324 mg].

-Procainamide (Procan, Procanbid)

IV: 15 mg/kg IV loading dose at 20 mg/min, followed by 2-4 mg/min continuous IV infusion.

PO: 500 mg (nonsustained release) PO q2h x 2 doses, then Procanbid 1-2 gm PO q12h [500, 1000 mg].

-Disopyramide (Nor-pace, Norpace CR) 100-300 mg PO q6-8h [100, 150, mg] or disopyramide CR 100-150 mg PO bid [100, 150 mg].

Class Ib:

-Lidocaine (Xylocaine) 75-100 mg IV, then 2-4 mg/min IV

-Mexiletine (Mexitil) 100-200 mg PO q8h, max 1200 mg/d [150, 200, 250 mg].

-Tocainide (Tonocard) loading 400-600 mg PO, then 400-600 mg PO q8-12h (1200-1800 mg/d) PO in divided doses q8-12h [400, 600 mg].

-Phenytoin (Dilantin), loading dose 100-300 mg IV given as 50 mg in NS over 10 min IV q5min, then 100 mg IV q5min prn.

Class Ic:

-Flecainide (Tambocor) 50-100 mg PO q12h, max 400 mg/d [50, 100, 150 mg].

-Propafenone (Rythmol) 150-300 mg PO q8h, max 1200 mg/d [150, 225, 300 mg].

Class II:

-Propranolol (Inderal) 1-3 mg IV in NS (max 0.15 mg/kg) or 20-80 mg PO tid-qid [10, 20, 40, 60, 80 mg]; propranolol-LA (Inderal-LA), 80-120 mg PO qd [60, 80, 120, 160 mg]

-Esmolol (Brevibloc) loading dose 500 mcg/kg over 1 min, then 50-200 mcg/kg/min IV infusion

-Atenolol (Tenormin) 50-100 mg/d PO [25, 50, 100 mg].

-Nadolol (Corgard) 40-100 mg PO qd-bid [20, 40, 80, 120, 160 mg].

-Metoprolol (Lopressor) 50-100 mg PO bid-tid [50, 100 mg], or metoprolol XL 50-200 mg PO qd [50, 100, 200 mg].

Class III:

-Amiodarone (Cordarone), PO loading 400-1200 mg/d in divided doses for 2-4 weeks, then 200-400 mg PO qd (5-10 mg/kg) [200 mg] or amiodarone (Cordarone) 150 mg in 100 mL of D5W, IV infusion over 10 min, then 900 mg in 500 mL of D5W, at 1 mg/min for 6 hrs, then at 0.5 mg/min thereafter.

-Bretylium (Bretylol) 5-10 mg/kg IV over 5-10 min, then maintenance of 1-4 mg/min IV or repeat boluses 5-10 mg/kg IV q6-8h; infusion of 1-4 mg/min IV.

-Sotalol (Betapace) 40-80 mg PO bid, max 320 mg/d in 2-3 divided doses [80, 160 mg].

4. **Extras:** CXR, ECG, Holter monitor, signal averaged ECG, cardiology consult.
5. **Labs:** SMA 7&12, Mg, calcium, CBC, drug levels. UA.

Hypertensive Emergency

1. **Admit to:**
2. **Diagnosis:** Hypertensive emergency
3. **Condition:**
4. **Vital signs:** q30min until BP controlled, then q4h.
5. **Activity:** Bed rest
6. **Nursing:** Intra-arterial BP monitoring, daily weights, inputs and outputs.
7. **Diet:** Clear liquids.
8. **IV Fluids:** D5W at TKO.
9. **Special Medications:**
   -Nitroprusside sodium 0.25-10 mcg/kg/min IV (50 mg in 250 mL of D5W), titrate to desired BP
   -Labetalol (Trandate, Normodyne) 20 mg IV bolus (0.25 mg/kg), then 20-80 mg boluses IV q10-15min titrated to desired BP. Infusion of 1.0-2.0 mg/min
   -Fenoldopam (Corlopam) 0.01mcg/kg/min IV infusion. Adjust dose by 0.025-0.05 mcg/kg/min q15min to max 0.3 mcg/kg/min. [10 mg in 250 mL D5W].
   -Nicardipine (Cardene IV) 5 mg/hr IV infusion, increase rate by 2.5 mg/hr every 15 min up to 15 mg/hr (25 mg in D5W 250 mL).
   -Enalaprilat (Vasotec IV) 1.25- 5.0 mg IV q6h. Do not use in presence of AMI.
   -Esmolol (Brevibloc) 500 mcg/kg/min IV infusion for 1 minute, then 50 mcg/kg/min; titrate by 50 mcg/kg/min increments to 300 mcg/kg/min (2.5 gm in D5W 250 mL).
   -Clonidine (Catapres), initial 0.1-0.2 mg PO followed by 0.05-0.1 mg per hour until DBP <115 (max total dose of 0.8 mg).
   -Phentolamine (pheochromocytoma), 5-10 mg IV, repeated as needed up to 20 mg.
   -Trimethaphan camsylate (Arfonad)(dissecting aneurysm) 2-4 mg/min IV infusion (500 mg in 500 mL of D5W).
10. **Symptomatic Medications:**
11. **Extras:** Portable CXR, ECG, echocardiogram.
12. **Labs:** CBC, SMA 7, UA with micro. TSH, free T4, 24h urine for metanephrines. Plasma catecholamines, urine drug screen.

Hypertension

I. **Initial Diagnostic Evaluation of Hypertension**
   A. **15 Lead electrocardiography** may document evidence of ischemic heart disease, rhythm and conduction disturbances, or left ventricular hypertrophy.
   B. **Screening labs** include a complete blood count, glucose, potassium, calcium, creatinine, BUN, uric acid, and fasting lipid panel.
   C. **Urinalysis.** Dipstick testing should include glucose, protein, and hemoglobin.

D. Selected patients may require plasma renin activity, 24 hour urine catecholamines, or renal function testing (glomerular filtration rate and blood flow).

II. Antihypertensive Drugs

A. Thiazide Diuretics

1. **Hydrochlorothiazide (HCTZ, HydroDiuril),** 12.5-25 mg qd [25 mg].
2. **Chlorothiazide (Diuril)** 250 mg qd [250, 500 mg].
3. **Thiazide/Potassium Sparing Diuretic Combinations**
   a. **Maxzide** (hydrochlorothiazide 50/triamterene 75 mg) 1 tab qd.
   b. **Moduretic** (hydrochlorothiazide 50 mg/amiloride 5 mg) 1 tab qd.
   c. **Dyazide** (hydrochlorothiazide 25 mg/triamterene 37.5) 1 cap qd.

B. Beta-Adrenergic Blockers

1. **Cardioselective Beta-Blockers**
   a. **Atenolol (Tenormin)** initial dose 50 mg qd, then 50-100 mg qd, max 200 mg/d [25, 50, 100 mg].
   b. **Metoprolol XL (Toprol XL)** 100-200 mg qd [50, 100, 200 mg tab ER].
   c. **Bisoprolol (Zebeta)** 2.5-10 mg qd; max 20 mg qd [5,10 mg].
2. **Non-Cardioselective Beta-Blockers**
   a. **Propranolol LA (Inderal LA),** 80-160 mg qd [60, 80, 120, 160 mg].
   b. **Nadolol (Corgard)** 40-80 mg qd, max 320 mg/d [20, 40, 80, 120, 160 mg].
   c. **Pindolol (Visken)** 5-20 mg qd, max 60 mg/d [5, 10 mg].
   d. **Carteolol (Cartrol)** 2.5-10 mg qd [2.5, 5 mg].

C. Angiotensin-Converting Enzyme (ACE) Inhibitors

1. **Ramipril (Altace)** 2.5-10 mg qd, max 20 mg/day [1.25, 2.5, 5, 10 mg].
2. **Quinapril (Accupril)** 20-80 mg qd [5, 10, 20, 40 mg].
3. **Lisinopril (Zestril, Prinivil)** 10-40 mg qd [2.5, 5, 10, 20, 40 mg].
4. **Benazepril (Lotensin)** 10-40 mg qd, max 80 mg/day [5, 10, 20, 40 mg].
5. **Fosinopril (Monopril)** 10-40 mg qd [10, 20 mg].
6. **Enalapril (Vasotec)** 5-40 mg qd, max 40 mg/day [2.5, 5, 10, 20 mg].
7. **Moexipril (Univasc)** 7.5-15 mg qd [7.5 mg].

D. Angiotensin Receptor Antagonists

1. **Losartan (Cozaar)** 25-50 mg bid [25, 50 mg].
2. **Valsartan (Diovan)** 80-160 mg qd; max 320 mg qd [80, 160 mg].
3. **Irbesartan (Avapro)** 150 mg qd; max 300 mg qd [75, 150, 300 mg].
4. **Candesartan (Atacand)** 8-16 mg qd-bid [4, 8, 16, 32 mg].
5. **Telmisartan (Micardis)** 40-80 mg qd [40, 80 mg].

E. Calcium Entry Blockers

1. **Diltiazem SR (Cardizem SR)** 60-120 mg bid [60, 90, 120 mg] or **Cardizem CD** 180-360 mg qd [120, 180, 240, 300 mg].
2. **Nifedipine XL (Procardia-XL, Adalat-CC)** 30-90 mg qd [30, 60, 90 mg].
3. **Verapamil SR (Calan SR, Covera-HS)** 120-240 mg qd [120, 180, 240 mg].
4. **Amlodipine (Norvasc)** 2.5-10 mg qd [2.5, 5, 10 mg].

5. **Felodipine (Plendil)** 5-10 mg qd [2.5, 5, 10 mg].

Syncope

1. **Admit to:** Monitored ward
2. **Diagnosis:** Syncope
3. **Condition:**
4. **Vital signs:** q1h, postural BP and pulse q12h. Call physician if BP >160/90, <90/60; P >120, <50; R>25, <10
5. **Activity:** Bed rest.
6. **Nursing:** Fingerstick glucose.
7. **Diet:** Regular
8. **IV Fluids:** Normal saline at TKO.
9. **Special medications:**

High-grade AV Block with Syncope:

-Atropine 1 mg IV x 2.

-Isoproterenol 0.5-1 mcg/min initially, then slowly titrate to 10 mcg/min IV infusion (1 mg in 250 mL NS).

-Transthoracic pacing.

Drug-induced Syncope:

-Discontinue vasodilators, centrally acting hypotensive agents, tranquilizers, antidepressants, and alcohol use.

Vasovagal Syncope:

-Scopolamine 1.5 mg transdermal patch q3 days.

Postural Syncope:

-Midodrine (ProAmatine) 2.5 mg PO tid, then increase to 5-10 mg PO tid [2.5, 5 mg]; contraindicated in coronary artery disease.

-Fludrocortisone 0.1-1.0 mg PO qd.

10. **Extras:** CXR, ECG, 24h Holter monitor, electrophysiologic study, tilt test, CT/MRI, EEG, echocardiogram.
11. **Labs:** CBC, SMA 7&12, CK-MB, troponin T, Mg, calcium, drug levels. UA, urine drug screen.

Pulmonary Disorders

Asthma

1. **Admit to:**
2. **Diagnosis:** Exacerbation of asthma
3. **Condition:**
4. **Vital signs:** q6h. Call physician if P >140; R >30, <10; T >38.5°C; pulse oximeter <90%
5. **Activity:** Up as tolerated.
6. **Nursing:** Pulse oximeter, bedside peak flow rate before and after bronchodilator treatments.
7. **Diet:** Regular, no caffeine.
8. **IV Fluids:** D5 ½ NS at 125 cc/h.
9. **Special Medications:**
   -Oxygen 2 L/min by NC. Keep O_2 sat >90%.

Beta Agonists, Acute Treatment:

-Albuterol (Ventolin) 0.5 mg and ipratropium (Atrovent) 0.5 mg in 2.5 mL NS q1-2h until peak flow meter ≥200-250 L/min and sat ≥90%, then q4h **OR**

-Albuterol (Ventolin) MDI 3-8 puffs, then 2 puffs q3-6h prn, or powder 200 mcg/capsule inhaled qid.

-Albuterol/Ipratropium (Combivent) 2-4 puffs qid.

Systemic Corticosteroids:

-Methylprednisolone (Solu-Medrol) 60-125 mg IV q6h; then 30-60 mg PO qd. **OR**

-Prednisone 20-60 mg PO qAM.

Aminophylline and Theophylline (second-line therapy):

-Aminophylline load dose: 5.6 mg/kg **total** body weight in 100 mL D5W IV over 20min. Maintenance of 0.5-0.6 mg/kg **ideal** body weight/h (500 mg in 250 mL D5W); reduce if elderly, heart/liver failure (0.2-0.4 mg/kg/hr). Reduce load 50-75% if taking theophylline (1 mg/kg of aminophylline will raise levels 2 mcg/mL) **OR**

-Theophylline IV solution loading dose 4.5 mg/kg **total** body weight, then 0.4-0.5 mg/kg **ideal** body weight/hr.

-Theophylline (Theo-Dur) PO loading dose of 6 mg/kg, then maintenance of 100-400 mg PO bid-tid (3 mg/kg q8h); 80% of total daily IV aminophylline in 2-3 doses.

Inhaled Corticosteroids (adjunct therapy):

-Beclomethasone (Beclovent) MDI 4-8 puffs bid, with spacer 5 min after bronchodilator, followed by gargling with water

-Triamcinolone (Azmacort) MDI 2 puffs tid-qid or 4 puffs bid.

-Flunisolide (AeroBid) MDI 2-4 puffs bid.

-Fluticasone (Flovent) 2-4 puffs bid (44 or 110 mcg/puff); requires 1-2 weeks for full effect.

Maintenance Treatment:

-Salmeterol (Serevent) 2 puffs bid; not effective for acute asthma because of delayed onset of action.

-Pirbuterol (Maxair) MDI 2 puffs q4-6h prn.

-Bitolterol (Tornalate) MDI 2-3 puffs q1-3min, then 2-3 puffs q4-8h prn.

-Fenoterol (Berotec) MDI 3 puffs, then 2 bid-qid.

-Ipratropium (Atrovent) MDI 2-3 puffs tid-qid.

Prevention and Prophylaxis:

-Cromolyn (Intal) 2-4 puffs tid-qid.

-Nedocromil (Tilade) 2-4 puffs bid-qid.

-Montelukast (Singulair) 10 mg PO qd.

-Zafirlukast (Accolate) 20 mg PO bid.

-Zileuton (Zyflo) 600 mg PO qid.

Acute Bronchitis

-Ampicillin/sulbactam (Unasyn) 1.5 gm IV q6h **OR**

-Ampicillin 0.5-1 gm IV q6h or 250-500 mg PO qid **OR**

-Cefuroxime (Zinacef) 750 mg IV q8h **OR**

-Cefuroxime axetil (Ceftin) 250-500 mg PO bid **OR**

-Trimethoprim/Sulfamethoxazole (Bactrim DS), 1 tab PO bid **OR**

-Levofloxacin (Levaquin) 500 mg PO/IV PO qd [250, 500 mg].

10. Symptomatic Medications:

-Docusate sodium (Colace) 100 mg PO qhs.

-Ranitidine (Zantac) 50 mg IV q8h or 150 mg PO bid.

11. Extras: Portable CXR, ECG, pulmonary function tests before and after bronchodilators; pulmonary rehabilitation.

12. Labs: ABG, CBC with eosinophil count, SMA7. Theophylline level stat and after 24h of infusion. Sputum Gram stain, C&S.

Chronic Obstructive Pulmonary Disease

1. **Admit to:**
2. **Diagnosis:** Exacerbation of COPD
3. **Condition:**
4. **Vital signs:** q4h. Call physician if P >130; R >30, <10; T >38.5°C; O_2 Sat <90%.
5. **Activity:** Up as tolerated; bedside commode.
6. **Nursing:** Pulse oximeter. Measure peak flow with portable peak flow meter bid and chart with vital signs. No sedatives.
7. **Diet:** No added salt, no caffeine. Push fluids.
8. **IV Fluids:** D5 ½ NS with 20 mEq KCL/L at 125 cc/h.
9. **Special Medications:**

-Oxygen 1-2 L/min by NC or 24-35% by Venturi mask, keep O_2 saturation 90-91%.

Beta-Agonists, Acute Treatment:

-Albuterol (Ventolin) 0.5 mg and ipratropium (Atrovent) 0.5 mg in 2.5 mL NS q1-2h until peak flow meter ≥200-250 L/min, then q4h **OR**

-Albuterol (Ventolin) MDI 2-4 puffs q4-6h.
-Albuterol/Ipratropium (Combivent) 2-4 puffs qid.

Corticosteroids and Anticholinergics:

-Methylprednisolone (Solu-Medrol) 60-125 mg IV q6h or 30-60 mg PO qd.
Followed by:
-Prednisone 20-60 mg PO qd.
-Triamcinolone (Azmacort) MDI 2 puffs qid or 4 puffs bid.
-Beclomethasone (Beclovent) MDI 4-8 puffs bid with spacer, followed by gargling with water **OR**
-Flunisolide (AeroBid) MDI 2-4 puffs bid **OR**
-Ipratropium (Atrovent) MDI 2 puffs tid-qid **OR**
-Fluticasone (Flovent) 2-4 puffs bid (44 or 110 mcg/puff.

Aminophylline and Theophylline (second line therapy):

-Aminophylline loading dose, 5.6 mg/kg **total** body weight over 20 min (if not already on theophylline); then 0.5-0.6 mg/kg **ideal** body weight/hr (500 mg in 250 mL of D5W); reduce if elderly, or heart or liver disease (0.2-0.4 mg/kg/hr). Reduce loading to 50-75% if already taking theophylline (1 mg/kg of aminophylline will raise levels by 2 mcg/mL) **OR**
-Theophylline IV solution loading dose, 4.5 mg/kg **total** body weight, then 0.4-0.5 mg/kg **ideal** body weight/hr.
-Theophylline long acting (Theo-Dur) 100-400 mg PO bid-tid (3 mg/kg q8h); 80% of daily IV aminophylline in 2-3 doses.

Acute Bronchitis

-Ampicillin 1 gm IV q6h or 500 mg PO qid **OR**
-Trimethoprim/sulfamethoxazole (Septra DS) 160/800 mg PO bid or 160/800 mg IV q12h (10-15 mL in 100 cc D5W tid) **OR**
-Cefuroxime (Zinacef) 750 mg IV q8h **OR**
-Ampicillin/sulbactam (Unasyn) 1.5 gm IV q6h **OR**
-Doxycycline (Vibra-tabs) 100 mg PO/IV bid
-Azithromycin (Zithromax) 500 mg x 1, then 250 mg PO qd x 4 or 500 mg IV q24h **OR**
-Clarithromycin (Biaxin) 250-500 mg PO bid **OR**
-Levofloxacin (Levaquin) 500 mg PO/IV qd [250, 500 mg] **OR**
-Sparfloxacin (Zagam) 400 mg PO x 1, then 200 mg PO qd [200 mg].

10. Symptomatic Medications:

-Docusate sodium (Colace) 100 mg PO qhs.
-Ranitidine (Zantac)150 mg PO bid or 50 mg IV q8h.

11. Extras: Portable CXR, PFT's with bronchodilators, ECG.

12. Labs: ABG, CBC, SMA7, UA. Theophylline level stat and after 12-24h of infusion. Sputum Gram stain and C&S, alpha 1 antitrypsin level.

Hemoptysis

1. **Admit to:** Intensive care unit
2. **Diagnosis:** Hemoptysis
3. **Condition:**
4. **Vital signs:** q1-6h. Orthostatic BP and pulse bid. Call physician if BP >160/90, <90/60; P >130, <50; R>25, <10; T >38.5°C; O_2 sat <90%
5. **Activity:** Bed rest with bedside commode. Keep patient in lateral decubitus, Trendelenburg's position, bleeding side down.
6. **Nursing:** Quantify all sputum and expectorated blood, suction prn. O_2 at 100% by mask, pulse oximeter. Discontinue narcotics and sedatives. Have double lumen endotracheal tube available for use.
7. **Diet:**
8. **IV Fluids:** 1 L of NS wide open (≥6 gauge), then transfuse PRBC, Foley to gravity.
9. **Special Medications:**
   -Transfuse 2-4 U PRBC wide open.
   -Promethazine/codeine (Phenergan with codeine) 5 cc PO q4-6h prn cough. Contraindicated in massive hemoptysis.
   -Consider empiric antibiotics if any suggestion that bronchitis or infection may be contributing to hemoptysis.

10. Extras: CXR PA, LAT, ECG, VQ scan, contrast CT, bronchoscopy. PPD, pulmonary and thoracic surgery consults.

11. Labs: Type and cross 2-4 U PRBC. ABG, CBC, platelets, SMA7 and 12, ESR. Anti-glomerular basement antibody, rheumatoid factor, complement, anti-nuclear cytoplasmic antibody. Sputum Gram stain, C&S, AFB, fungal culture, and cytology qAM for 3 days. UA, INR/PTT, von Willebrand Factor. Repeat CBC q6h.

Anaphylaxis

1. **Admit to:**
2. **Diagnosis:** Anaphylaxis
3. **Condition:**
4. **Vital signs:** q1h; Call physician if BP systolic >160, <90; diastolic. >90, <60; P >120, <50; R>25, <10; T >38.5°C
5. **Activity:** Bedrest
6. **Nursing:** O_2 at 6 L/min by NC or mask. Keep patient in Trendelenburg's position, No. 4 or 5 endotracheal tube at bedside.
7. **Diet:** NPO
8. **IV Fluids:** 2 IV lines. Normal saline or LR 1 L over 1-2h, then D5 ½ NS at 125 cc/h. Foley to closed drainage.
9. **Special Medications:**

Gastrointestinal Decontamination:

-Gastric lavage if indicated for recent oral ingestion.
-Activated charcoal 50-100 gm, followed by cathartic.

Bronchodilators:

-Epinephrine (1:1000) 0.3-0.5 mL SQ or IM q10min or 1-4 mcg/min IV **OR** in severe life threatening reactions, give 0.5 mg (5.0 mL of 1: 10,000 sln) IV q5-10min prn. Epinephrine, 0.3 mg of 1:1000 sln may be injected SQ at site of allergen injection **OR**

-Albuterol (Ventolin) 0.5%, 0.5 mL in 2.5 mL NS q30min by nebulizer prn **OR**

-Aerosolized 2% racemic epinephrine 0.5-0.75 mL.

Corticosteroids:

-Methylprednisolone (Solu-Medrol) 250 mg IV x 1, then 125 mg IV q6h **OR**

-Hydrocortisone sodium succinate 200 mg IV x 1, then 100 mg q6h, followed by oral prednisone 60 mg PO qd, tapered over 5 days.

Antihistamines:

-Diphenhydramine (Benadryl) 25-50 mg IV q4-6h **OR**

-Hydroxyzine (Vistaril) 25-50 mg IM or PO q2-4h.

-Cimetidine (Tagamet) 300 mg IV or PO q6h **OR**

-Ranitidine (Zantac) 150 mg IV or PO bid.

Pressors and other Agents:

-Norepinephrine (Levophed) 8-12 mcg/min IV, titrate to systolic 100 mmHg (8 mg in 500 mL D5W) **OR**

-Isoproterenol (Isuprel) 0.5-5 mcg/min IV **OR**

-Dopamine (Intropin) 5-20 mcg/kg/min IV.

10. **Extras:** Portable CXR, ECG, allergy/immunology consult.
11. **Labs:** CBC, SMA 7&12.

Pleural Effusion

1. **Admit to:**
2. **Diagnosis:** Pleural effusion
3. **Condition:**
4. **Vital signs:** q shift. Call physician if BP >160/90, <90/60; P>120, <50; R>25, <10; T >38.5°C
5. **Activity:**
6. **Diet:** Regular.
7. **IV Fluids:** D5W at TKO
8. **Extras:** CXR PA and LAT, repeat after thoracentesis; left and right lateral decubitus x-rays, ECG, ultrasound, PPD; pulmonary consult.
9. **Labs:** CBC, SMA 7&12, protein, albumin, amylase, ANA, ESR, INR/PTT, UA. Cryptococcal antigen, histoplasma antigen, fungal culture.

Thoracentesis:

Tube 1: LDH, protein, amylase, triglyceride, glucose (10 mL).

Tube 2: Gram stain, C&S, AFB, fungal C&S (20-60 mL, heparinized).

Tube 3: Cell count and differential (5-10 mL, EDTA).

Syringe: pH (2 mL collected anaerobically, heparinized on ice)

Bag or Bottle: Cytology.

Hematologic Disorders

Anticoagulant Overdose

Unfractionated Heparin Overdose:

1. Discontinue heparin infusion.
2. Protamine sulfate, 1 mg IV for every 100 units of heparin infused in preceding hour, dilute in 25 mL fluid IV over 10 min (max 50 mg in 10 min period). Watch for signs of anaphylaxis, especially if patient has been on NPH insulin therapy.

Low Molecular Weight Heparin (Enoxaparin) Overdose:

-Protamine sulfate 1 mg IV for each 1 mg of enoxaparin given. Repeat protamine 0.5 mg IV for each 1 mg of enoxaparin, if bleeding continues after 2-4 hours. Measure factor Xa.

Warfarin (Coumadin) Overdose:

-Gastric lavage and activated charcoal if recent oral ingestion. Discontinue Coumadin and heparin, and monitor hematocrit q2h.

Partial Reversal:

-Vitamin K (Phytonadione), 0.5-1.0 mg IV/SQ. Check INR in 24 hours, and repeat vitamin K dose if INR remains elevated.

Minor Bleeds:

-Vitamin K (Phytonadione), 5-10 mg IV/SQ q12h, titrated to desired INR.

Serious Bleeds:

-Vitamin K (Phytonadione), 10-20 mg in 50-100 mL fluid IV over 30-60 min (check INR q6h until corrected) **AND**

-Fresh frozen plasma 2-4 units x 1.

-Type and cross match for 2 units of PRBC, and transfuse wide open.

-Cryoprecipitate 10 U x 1 if fibrinogen is less than100 mg/dL.

Labs: CBC, platelets, PTT, INR.

Deep Venous Thrombosis

1. **Admit to:**
2. **Diagnosis:** Deep vein thrombosis
3. **Condition:**
4. **Vital signs:** q shift. Call physician if BP systolic >160, <90 diastolic, >90, <60; P >120, <50; R>25, <10; T >38.5°C.
5. **Activity:** Bed rest with legs elevated.
6. **Nursing:** Guaiac stools, warm packs to leg prn; measure calf circumference qd; no intramuscular injections.
7. **Diet:** Regular
8. **IV Fluids:** D5W at TKO

9. Special Medications:
Anticoagulation:
- -Heparin (unfractionated) IV bolus 5000-10,000 Units (100 U/kg) IVP, then 1000-1500 U/h IV infusion (20 U/kg/h) [25,000 U in 500 mL D5W (50 U/mL)]. Check PTT 6 hours after initial bolus; adjust q6h until PTT 1.5-2.0 times control (50-80 sec). Overlap heparin and warfarin (Coumadin) for at least 4 days and discontinue heparin when INR has been 2.0-3.0 for two consecutive days.
- -Enoxaparin (Lovenox) 1 mg/kg SQ q12h. Overlap enoxaparin and warfarin as outlined above.
- -Warfarin (Coumadin) 5-10 mg PO qd x 2-3 d; maintain INR 2.0-3.0. Coumadin is initiated on the first or second day only if the PTT is 1.5-2.0 times control [tab 1, 2, 2.5, 3, 4, 5, 6, 7.5, 10 mg].

10. Symptomatic Medications:
- -Propoxyphene/acetaminophen (Darvocet N100) 1-2 tab PO q3-4h prn pain **OR**
- -Hydrocodone/acetaminophen (Vicodin), 1-2 tab q4-6h PO prn pain.
- -Docusate sodium (Colace) 100 mg PO qhs.
- -Ranitidine (Zantac) 150 mg PO bid.

11. Extras: CXR PA and LAT, ECG; Doppler scan of legs, venography. V/Q scan. Lower extremity (venogram).

12. Labs: CBC, INR/PTT, SMA 7. Protein C, protein S, antithrombin III, anticardiolipin antibody. UA with dipstick for blood. PTT 6h after bolus and q4-6h until PTT 1.5-2.0 x control then qd. INR at initiation of warfarin and qd.

Pulmonary Embolism

1. **Admit to:**
2. **Diagnosis:** Pulmonary embolism
3. **Condition:**
4. **Vital signs:** q1-4h. Call physician if BP >160/90, <90/60; P >120, <50; R >30, <10; T >38.5°C; O_2 sat < 90%
5. **Activity:** Bedrest with bedside commode
6. **Nursing:** Pulse oximeter, guaiac stools, O_2 at 2 L by NC. Antiembolism stockings. No intramuscular injections.
7. **Diet:** Regular
8. **IV Fluids:** D5W at TKO.
9. **Special Medications:**

Anticoagulation:
- -Heparin IV bolus 5000-10,000 Units (100 U/kg) IVP, then 1000-1500 U/h IV infusion (20 U/kg/h) [25,000 U in 500 mL D5W (50 U/mL)]. Check PTT 6 hours after initial bolus; adjust q6h until PTT to 1.5-2 times control (60-80 sec). Overlap heparin and Coumadin for at least 4 days and discontinue heparin when INR has been 2.0-3.0 for two consecutive days.
- -Enoxaparin (Lovenox) 1 mg/kg sq q12h for 5 days for uncomplicated pulmonary embolism. Overlap warfarin as outlined above.

-Warfarin (Coumadin) 5-10 mg PO qd for 2-3 d, then 2-5 mg PO qd. Maintain INR of 2.0-3.0. Coumadin is initiated on second day if the PTT is 1.5-2.0 times control. Check INR at initiation of warfarin and qd [tab 1, 2, 2.5, 3, 4, 5, 6, 7.5, 10 mg].

Thrombolytics (indicated if hemodynamic compromise):

Baseline Labs: CBC, INR/PTT, fibrinogen q6h.

Alteplase (recombinant tissue plasminogen activator, Activase): 100 mg IV infusion over 2 hours, followed by heparin infusion at 15 U/kg/h to maintain PTT 1.5-2.5 x control **OR**

Streptokinase (Streptase): Pretreat with methylprednisolone 250 mg IV push and diphenhydramine (Benadryl) 50 mg IV push. Then give streptokinase, 250,000 units IV over 30 min, then 100,000 units/h for 24-72 hours. Initiate heparin infusion at 10 U/kg/hour; maintain PTT 1.5-2.5 x control.

10. Symptomatic Medications:

-Meperidine (Demerol) 25-100 mg IV prn pain.

-Docusate sodium (Colace) 100 mg PO qhs.

-Ranitidine (Zantac) 150 mg PO bid.

11. Extras: CXR PA and LAT, ECG, VQ scan; pulmonary angiography; Doppler scan of lower extremities.

12. Labs: CBC, INR/PTT, SMA7, ABG, cardiac enzymes. Protein C, protein S, antithrombin III, anticardiolipin antibody. UA . PTT 6 hours after bolus and q4-6h. INR at initiation of warfarin and qd.

Sickle Cell Crisis

1. **Admit to:**
2. **Diagnosis:** Sickle Cell Crisis
3. **Condition:**
4. **Vital signs:** q shift.
5. **Activity:** Bedrest
6. **Nursing:**
7. **Diet:** Regular diet, push oral fluids.
8. **IV Fluids:** D5 ½ NS at 100-125 mL/h.
9. **Special Medications:**

-Oxygen 2 L/min by NC or 30-100% by mask.

-Meperidine (Demerol) 50-150 mg IM/IV/SC q4-6h prn pain.

-Hydroxyzine (Vistaril) 25-100 mg IM/IV/PO q3-4h prn pain.

-Morphine sulfate 10 mg IV/IM/SC q2-4h prn pain **OR**

-Ketorolac (Toradol) 30-60 mg IV/IM then 15-30 mg IV/IM q6h prn pain (maximum of 5 days).

-Acetaminophen/codeine (Tylenol 3) 1-2 tabs PO q4-6h prn.

-Folic acid 1 mg PO qd.

-Penicillin V (prophylaxis), 250 mg PO qid [tabs 125,250,500 mg].

-Prochlorperazine (Compazine) 5-10 mg PO or IM q6h prn nausea or vomiting.

Vaccination:

-Pneumovax before discharge 0.5 cc IM x 1 dose.

-Influenza vaccine (Fluogen) 0.5 cc IM once a year in the Fall.

10. Extras: CXR.

11. Labs: CBC, SMA 7, blood C&S, reticulocyte count, blood type and screen, parvovirus titers. UA.

Infectious Diseases

Meningitis

1. **Admit to:**
2. **Diagnosis:** Meningitis.
3. **Condition:**
4. **Vital signs:** q1h. Call physician if BP systolic >160/90, <90/60; P >120, <50; R>25, <10; T >39°C or less than 36°C
5. **Activity:** Bed rest with bedside commode.
6. **Nursing:** Respiratory isolation, inputs and outputs, lumbar puncture tray at bedside.
7. **Diet:** NPO
8. **IV Fluids:** D5 ½ NS at 125 cc/h with KCL 20 mEq/L.
9. **Special Medications:**

Empiric Therapy 15-50 years old:

-Vancomycin 1 gm IV q12h **AND EITHER**

-Ceftriaxone (Rocephin) 2 gm IV q12h (max 4 gm/d) **OR**
Cefotaxime (Claforan) 2 gm IV q4h.

Empiric Therapy >50 years old, Alcoholic, Corticosteroids or Hematologic Malignancy or other Debilitating Condition:

-Ampicillin 2 gm IV q4h **AND EITHER**

-Cefotaxime (Claforan) 2 gm IV q6h **OR**
Ceftriaxone (Rocephin) 2 gm IV q12h **OR**
Ceftazidime (Fortaz) 2 gm IV q8h.

-Use Vancomycin 1 mg IV q12h in place of ampicillin if drug-resistant pneumococcus is suspected.

10. **Symptomatic Medications:**

-Acetaminophen (Tylenol) 650 mg PO/PR q4-6h prn temp >39°C.

11. **Extras:** CXR, ECG, PPD, CT scan.
12. **Labs:** CBC, SMA 7&12. Blood C&S x 2. UA with micro, urine C&S. Antibiotic levels peak and trough after 3rd dose, VDRL.

Lumbar Puncture:

CSF Tube 1: Gram stain, C&S for bacteria (1-4 mL).

CSF Tube 2: Glucose, protein (1-2 mL).

CSF Tube 3: Cell count and differential (1-2 mL).

CSF Tube 4: Latex agglutination or counterimmunoelectrophoresis antigen tests for S. pneumoniae, H. influenzae (type B), N. meningitides, E. coli, group B strep, VDRL, cryptococcal antigen, toxoplasma titers. India ink, fungal cultures, cryptococcal antigen, AFB (8-10 mL).

Infective Endocarditis

1. **Admit to:**
2. **Diagnosis:** Infective endocarditis
3. **Condition:**
4. **Vital signs:** q4h. Call physician if BP systolic >160/90, <90/60; P >120, <50; R>25, <10; T >38.5°C
5. **Activity:** Up ad lib
6. **Diet:** Regular
7. **IV Fluids:** Heparin lock with flush q shift.
8. **Special Medications:**

Subacute Bacterial Endocarditis Empiric Therapy:
-Penicillin G 3-5 million U IV q4h or ampicillin 2 gm IV q4h **AND**
Gentamicin 1-1.5/mg/kg IV q8h.

Acute Bacterial Endocarditis Empiric Therapy
-Gentamicin 2 mg/kg IV; then 1-1.5 mg/kg IV q8h **AND**
Nafcillin or oxacillin 2 gm IV q4h **OR**
Vancomycin 1 gm IV q12h (1 gm in 250 mL of D5W over 1h).

Streptococci viridans/bovis:
-Penicillin G 3-5 million U IV q4h for 4 weeks **OR**
Vancomycin 1 gm IV q12h for 4 weeks **AND**
Gentamicin 1 mg/kg q8h for first 2 weeks.

Enterococcus:
-Gentamicin 1 mg/kg IV q8h for 4-6 weeks **AND**
Ampicillin 2 gm IV q4h for 4-6 weeks **OR**
Vancomycin 1 gm IV q12h for 4-6 weeks.

Staphylococcus aureus (methicillin sensitive, native valve):
-Nafcillin or Oxacillin 2 gm IV q4h for 4-6 weeks **OR**
Vancomycin 1 gm IV q12h for 4-6 weeks **AND**
Gentamicin 1 mg/kg IV q8h for first 3-5 days.

Methicillin resistant Staphylococcus aureus (native valve):
-Vancomycin 1 gm IV q12h (1 gm in 250 mL D5W over 1h) for 4-6 weeks **AND**
Gentamicin 1 mg/kg IV q8h for 3-5 days.

Methicillin resistant Staph aureus or epidermidis (prosthetic valve):
-Vancomycin 1 gm IV q12h for 6 weeks **AND**
Rifampin 600 mg PO q8h for 6 weeks **AND**
Gentamicin 1 mg/kg IV q8h for 2 weeks.

Culture Negative Endocarditis:
-Penicillin G 3-5 million U IV q4h for 4-6 weeks **OR**
Ampicillin 2 gm IV q4h for 4-6 weeks **AND**
Gentamicin 1.5 mg/kg q8h for 2 weeks (or nafcillin, 2 gm IV q4h, and gentamicin if Staph aureus suspected in drug abuser or prosthetic valve).

Fungal Endocarditis:
-Amphotericin B 0.5 mg/kg/d IV plus flucytosine (5-FC) 150 mg/kg/d PO.

9. **Extras:** CXR PA and LAT, echocardiogram, ECG.
11. **Labs:** CBC with differential, SMA 7&12. Blood C&S x 3-4 over 24h, serum

cidal titers, minimum inhibitory concentration, minimum bactericidal concentration. Repeat C&S in 48h, then once a week. Antibiotic levels peak and trough at 3rd dose. UA, urine C&S.

Pneumonia

1. **Admit to:**
2. **Diagnosis:** Pneumonia
3. **Condition:**
4. **Vital signs:** q4-8h. Call physician if BP >160/90, <90/60; P >120, <50; R>25, <10; T >38.5°C or O_2 saturation <90%.
5. **Activity:**
6. **Nursing:** Pulse oximeter, inputs and outputs, nasotracheal suctioning prn, incentive spirometry.
7. **Diet:** Regular.
8. **IV Fluids:** IV D5 ½ NS at 125 cc/hr.
9. **Special Medications:**

-Oxygen by NC at 2-4 L/min, or 24-50% by Ventimask, or 100% by non-rebreather (reservoir) to maintain O_2 saturation >90%.

Moderately ill Patients Without Underlying Lung Disease from the Community:

-Cefuroxime (Zinacef) 0.75-1.5 gm IV q8h **OR**
Ampicillin/sulbactam (Unasyn) 1.5 gm IV q6h **AND EITHER**
-Erythromycin 500 mg IV/PO q6h **OR**
Clarithromycin (Biaxin) 500 mg PO bid **OR**
Azithromycin (Zithromax) 500 mg PO x 1, then 250 mg PO qd x 4 **OR**
Doxycycline (Vibramycin) 100 mg IV/PO q12h.

Moderately ill Patients With Recent Hospitalization or Debilitated Nursing Home Patient:

-Ceftazidime (Fortaz) 1-2 gm IV q8h **OR**
Cefepime (Maxipime) 1-2 gm IV q12h **OR**
Cefoperazone (Cefobid) 1-2 gm IV q8h **AND EITHER**
Gentamicin 1.5-2 mg/kg IV, then 1.0-1.5 mg/kg IV q8h or 7 mg/kg in 50 mL of D5W over 60 min IV q24h **OR**
Ciprofloxacin (Cipro) 400 mg IV q12h or 500 mg PO q12h **OR**
Levofloxacin (Levaquin) 500 mg IV/PO qd.

Critically ill Patients:

-Initial treatment should consist of a macrolide with 2 antipseudomonal agents for synergistic activity:
-Erythromycin 0.5-1.0 gm IV q6h **AND EITHER**
-Ceftazidime 1-2 gm q8h **OR**
Piperacillin/tazobactam (Zosyn) 3.75-4.50 gm IV q6h **OR**
Ticarcillin/clavulanate (Timentin) 3.1 gm IV q6h **OR**
Imipenem/cilastatin (Primaxin) 0.5-1.0 gm IV q6h **AND EITHER**
-Levofloxacin (Levaquin) 500 mg IV q24h **OR**
Ciprofloxacin (Cipro) 400 mg IV q12h **OR**

Tobramycin 2.0 mg/kg IV, then 1.5 mg/kg IV q8h or 7 mg/kg IV q24h **OR**
Trovafloxacin (Trovan) 300 mg IV x 1, then 200 mg IV q24h.

Aspiration Pneumonia (community acquired):

-Clindamycin (Cleocin) 600-900 mg IV q8h (with or without gentamicin or 3rd gen cephalosporin) **OR**

-Ampicillin/sulbactam (Unasyn) 1.5-3 gm IV q6h (with or without gentamicin or 3rd gen cephalosporin)

Aspiration Pneumonia (nosocomial):

-Tobramycin 2 mg/kg IV then 1.5 mg/kg IV q8h or 7 mg/kg in 50 mLs of D5W over 60 min IV q24h **OR**

Ceftazidime (Fortaz) 1-2 gm IV q8h **AND EITHER**

-Clindamycin (Cleocin) 600-900 mg IV q8h **OR**

Ampicillin/sulbactam or ticarcillin/clavulanate, or piperacillin/tazobactam or imipenem/cilastatin (see above).

10. **Symptomatic Medications:**

-Acetaminophen (Tylenol) 650 mg 2 tab PO q4-6h prn temp >38°C or pain.

-Docusate sodium (Colace) 100 mg PO qhs.

-Ranitidine (Zantac) 150 mg PO bid or 50 mg IV q8h.

-Heparin 5000 U SQ q12h.

11. **Extras:** CXR PA and LAT, ECG, PPD.

12. **Labs:** CBC with differential, SMA 7&12, ABG. Blood C&S x 2. Sputum Gram stain, C&S. Methenamine silver sputum stain (PCP); AFB smear/culture. Aminoglycoside levels peak and trough at 3rd dose. UA, urine culture.

Specific Therapy for Pneumonia

Pneumococcal Pneumonia:

-Ceftriaxone (Rocephin) 2 gm IV q12h **OR**

-Cefotaxime (Claforan) 2 gm IV q6h **OR**

-Erythromycin 500 mg IV q6h **OR**

-Vancomycin 1 gm IV q12h if drug resistance.

Staphylococcus aureus Pneumonia:

-Nafcillin 2 gm IV q4h **OR**

-Oxacillin 2 gm IV q4h.

Klebsiella pneumoniae Pneumonia:

-Gentamicin 1.5-2 mg/kg IV, then 1.0-1.5 mg/kg IV q8h or 7 mg/kg in 50 mL of D5W over 60 min IV q24h **AND**

Ceftizoxime (Cefizox) 1-2 gm IV q8h **OR**

Cefotaxime (Claforan) 1-2 gm IV q6h.

Methicillin-resistant staphylococcus aureus:

-Vancomycin 1 gm IV q12h.

Haemophilus influenzae:

-Ampicillin 1-2 gm IV q6h (beta-lactamase negative) **OR**

-Ampicillin/sulbactam (Unasyn) 1.5-3.0 gm q6h **OR**

-Cefuroxime (Zinacef) 1.5 gm IV q8h (beta-lactamase pos) **OR**

-Ceftizoxime (Cefizox) 1-2 gm IV q8h **OR**
-Ciprofloxacin (Cipro) 400 mg IV q12h **OR**
-Ofloxacin (Floxin) 400 mg IV q12h.
-Levofloxacin (Levaquin) 500 mg IV q24h.

Pseudomonas aeruginosa:
-Tobramycin 1.5-2.0 mg/kg IV, then 1.5-2.0 mg/kg IV q8h or 7 mg/kg in 50 mL of D5W over 60 min IV q24h **AND EITHER**
Piperacillin, Ticarcillin, Mezlocillin or Azlocillin 3 gm IV q4h **OR**
Ceftazidime 1-2 gm IV q8h.

Mycoplasma pneumoniae:
-Clarithromycin (Biaxin) 500 mg PO bid **OR**
-Azithromycin (Zithromax) 500 mg PO x 1, then 250 mg PO qd for 4 days **OR**
-Erythromycin 500 mg PO or IV q6h **OR**
-Doxycycline (Vibramycin) 100 mg PO/IV q12h **OR**
-Levofloxacin (Levaquin) 500 mg PO/IV q24h.

Legionella pneumoniae:
-Erythromycin 1.0 gm IV q6h **OR**
-Levofloxacin (Levaquin) 500 mg PO/IV q24h.
-Rifampin 600 mg PO qd may be added to erythromycin or levofloxacin.

Moraxella catarrhalis:
-Trimethoprim/sulfamethoxazole (Bactrim, Septra) one DS tab PO bid or 10 mL IV q12h **OR**
-Ampicillin/sulbactam (Unasyn) 1.5-3 gm IV q6h **OR**
-Cefuroxime (Zinacef) 0.75-1.5 gm IV q8h **OR**
-Erythromycin 500 mg IV q6h **OR**
-Levofloxacin (Levaquin) 500 mg PO/IV q24h.

Anaerobic Pneumonia:
-Penicillin G 2 MU IV q4h **OR**
-Clindamycin (Cleocin) 900 mg IV q8h **OR**
-Metronidazole (Flagyl) 500 mg IV q8h.

Pneumocystis Carinii Pneumonia

1. **Admit to:**
2. **Diagnosis:** PCP pneumonia
3. **Condition:**
4. **Vital signs:** q2-6h. Call physician if BP >160/90, <90/60; P >120, <50; R>25, <10; T >38.5°C; O_2 sat <90%
5. **Activity:**
6. **Nursing:** Pulse oximeter.
7. **Diet:** Regular, encourage fluids.
8. **IV Fluids:** D5 ½ NS at 100 cc/h.
9. **Special Medications:**

Pneumocystis Carinii Pneumonia:
-Oxygen at 2-4 L/min by NC or by mask.
-Trimethoprim/sulfamethoxazole (Bactrim, Septra) 15 mg of TMP/kg/day (20

mL in 250 mL of D5W IVPB q8h) for 21 days [inj: 80/400 mg per 5 mL].

-If severe PCP (PaO_2 <70 mmHg): add prednisone 40 mg PO bid for 5 days, then 40 mg qd for 5 days, then 20 mg once daily for 11 days **OR** Methylprednisolone (Solu-Medrol) 30 mg IV q12h for 5 days, then 30 mg IV qd for 5 days, then 15 mg IV qd for 11 days.

-Pentamidine (Pentam) 4 mg/kg IV qd for 21 days, with prednisone as above. Pentamidine is an alternative if inadequate response or intolerant to TMP-SMX.

Pneumocystis Carinii Prophylaxis (previous PCP or CD4 <200, or constitutional symptoms):

-Trimethoprim/SMX DS (160/800 mg) PO qd **OR**

-Pentamidine, 300 mg in 6 mL sterile water via Respirgard II nebulizer over 20-30 min q4 weeks **OR**

-Dapsone (DDS) 50 mg PO bid or 100 mg twice a week; contraindicated in G-6-PD deficiency.

Antiretroviral Therapy:

A. Combination therapy with 3 agents (two nucleoside analogs and a protease inhibitor) is recommended as initial therapy.

B. Nucleoside Analogs

1. Zidovudine (Retrovir, AZT) 200 mg tid (100, 200 mg caps, 50 mg/5 mL syrup).
2. Lamivudine (Epivir, 3TC) 150 mg twice daily [150 mg].
3. Didanosine (Videx, ddI) 200 mg bid for patients >60 kg; or 125 mg bid for patients <60 kg.[chewable tabs: 25, 50, 100, 150 mg; pwd 100, 167, 250 mg packets].
4. Stavudine (Zerit, D4T) 40 mg bid [15-mg, 20-mg, 30-mg and 40-mg capsules].
5. Zalcitabine (Hivid, ddC) 0.75 mg tid [0.375, 0.75].
6. Abacavir (Ziagen) 300 mg PO bid [300 mg, 20 mg/mL].

C. Protease Inhibitors

1. Indinavir (Crixivan) 800 mg tid [200, 400 mg].
2. Saquinavir (Invirase) 600 mg tid with a meal [Cap 200 mg].
3. Ritonavir (Norvir) 600 mg bid [100 mg, 80 mg/dL]
4. Nelfinavir (Viracept) 750 mg PO tid [250 mg].

D. Non-Nucleoside Reverse Transcriptase Inhibitors

1. Nevirapine (Viramune) 200 mg qd for 2 weeks, then bid [200 mg].
2. Delavirdine (U-90) 400 mg tid.
3. Efavirenz (Sustiva) 600 mg PO qd [50, 100, 200 mg].

Postexposure HIV Prophylaxis

A. The injury should be immediately washed and scrubbed with soap and water.

B. Zidovudine 200 mg PO tid and lamivudine (3TC) 150 mg PO bid, plus indinavir (Crixivan) 800 mg PO tid for highest risk exposures. Treatment is continued for one month.

Zidovudine-Induced Neutropenia/Ganciclovir-Induced Leucopenia

-Recombinant human granulocyte colony-stimulating factor (G-CSF, Filgrastim, Neupogen) 1-2 mcg/kg SQ qd until absolute neutrophil count 500-1000; indicated only if the patient's endogenous erythropoietin level is low.

10. Extras: CXR PA and LAT.

11. Labs: ABG, CBC, SMA 7&12. Blood C&S x 2. Sputum for Gram stain, C&S, AFB. Giemsa immunofluorescence for Pneumocystis. CD4 count, HIV RNA, VDRL, serum cryptococcal antigen, UA.

Opportunistic Infections in HIV Infected Patients

Oral Candidiasis:

-Fluconazole (Diflucan) acute: 100-200 mg PO qd **OR**

-Ketoconazole (Nizoral), acute: 400 mg PO qd **OR**

-Itraconazole (Sporanox) 200 mg PO qd **OR**

-Clotrimazole (Mycelex) troches 10 mg dissolved slowly in mouth 5 times/d.

Candida Esophagitis:

-Fluconazole (Diflucan) 200-400 mg PO qd for 14-21 days **OR**

-Ketoconazole (Nizoral) 200 mg PO bid.

-Itraconazole (Sporanox) 200 mg PO qd for 2 weeks.

Primary or Recurrent Mucocutaneous HSV

-Acyclovir (Zovirax), 200-400 mg PO 5 times a day for 10 days, or 5 mg/kg IV q8h **OR** in cases of acyclovir resistance, foscarnet, 40 mg/kg IV q8h for 21 days.

Herpes Simplex Encephalitis (or visceral disease):

-Acyclovir 10 mg/kg IV q8h for 10-21 days.

Herpes Varicella Zoster

-Acyclovir 10 mg/kg IV over 60 min q8h for 7-14 days **OR** 800 mg PO 5 times/d for 7-10 days **OR**

-Famciclovir (Famvir) 500 mg PO q8h for 7 days [500 mg] **OR**

-Valacyclovir (Valtrex) 1000 mg PO q8h for 7 days [500 mg] **OR**

-Foscarnet (Foscavir) 40 mg/kg IV q8h.

Cytomegalovirus Retinitis:

-Ganciclovir (Cytovene) 5 mg/kg IV (dilute in 100 mL D5W over 60 min) q12h for 14-21 days **OR**

-Foscarnet (Foscavir) 60 mg/kg IV q8h for 2-3 weeks **OR**

-Cidofovir (Vistide) 5 mg/kg IV over 60 min q week for 2 weeks. Administer probenecid, 2 g PO 3 hours prior to cidofovir, 1 g PO 2 hours after, and 1 g PO 8 hours after.

Suppressive Treatment for Cytomegalovirus Retinitis:

-Ganciclovir 5 mg/kg qd.

-Foscarnet (Foscavir) 90-120 mg IV qd **OR**

-Cidofovir (Vistide) 5 mg/kg IV over 60 min every 2 weeks with probenecid.

Acute Toxoplasmosis:

-Pyrimethamine 200 mg, then 50-75 mg qd, plus sulfadiazine 1.0-1.5 gm PO q6h, plus folinic acid 10 mg PO qd **OR**

-Atovaquone (Mepron) 750 mg PO tid.

Suppressive Treatment for Toxoplasmosis:

-Pyrimethamine 25-50 mg PO qd plus sulfadiazine 0.5-1.0 gm PO q6h plus folinic acid 5 mg PO qd **OR**

-Pyrimethamine 50 mg PO qd, plus clindamycin 300 mg PO qid, plus folinic acid 5 mg PO qd.

Cryptococcus Neoformans Meningitis:

-Amphotericin B 0.7-1.0 mg/kg/d IV; total dosage of 2 g, with or without 5-flucytosine 100 mg/kg PO qd in divided doses, followed by fluconazole (Diflucan) 400 mg PO qd or itraconazole (Sporanox) 200 mg PO bid 6-8 weeks

OR

-Fluconazole (Diflucan) 400-800 mg PO qd for 8-12 weeks

Suppressive Treatment of Cryptococcus:

-Fluconazole (Diflucan) 200 mg PO qd indefinitely.

Active Tuberculosis:

-Isoniazid (INH) 300 mg PO qd; and rifampin 600 mg PO qd; and pyrazinamide 15-25 mg/kg PO qd (500 mg bid-tid); and ethambutol 15-25 mg/kg PO qd (400 mg bid-tid).

-All four drugs are continued for 2 months; isoniazid and rifampin are continued for a period of at least 9 months and at least 6 months after the last negative cultures.

-Pyridoxine (Vitamin B6) 50 mg PO qd concurrent with INH.

Prophylaxis for Inactive Tuberculosis:

-Isoniazid 300 mg PO qd; and pyridoxine 50 mg PO qd for 12 months.

Disseminated Mycobacterium Avium Complex (MAC):

-Clarithromycin (Biaxin) 500 mg PO bid **AND**

Ethambutol 800-1000 mg qd; with or without rifabutin 450 mg qd.

Prophylaxis against MAC:

-Azithromycin (Zithromax) 1200 mg once a week.

Disseminated Coccidioidomycosis:

-Amphotericin B 0.5-0.8 mg/kg IV qd, to a total dose 2.0 gm **OR**

-Fluconazole (Diflucan) 400-800 mg PO or IV qd.

Disseminated Histoplasmosis:

-Amphotericin B 0.5-0.8 mg/kg IV qd, to a total dose 15 mg/kg **OR**

-Fluconazole (Diflucan) 400 mg PO qd. **OR**

-Itraconazole (Sporanox) 300 mg PO bid for 3 days, then 200 mg PO bid.

Suppressive Treatment for Histoplasmosis:

-Fluconazole (Diflucan) 400 mg PO qd **OR**

-Itraconazole (Sporanox) 200 mg PO bid.

Septic Arthritis

1. **Admit to:**
2. **Diagnosis:** Septic arthritis
3. **Condition:**
4. **Vital signs:** q shift
5. **Activity:** No weight bearing on infected joint. Up in chair as tolerated. Bedside commode with assistance.
6. **Nursing:** Warm compresses prn, keep joint immobilized. Passive range of

motion exercises of the affected joint bid; otherwise, keep knee in resting splint.

7. **Diet:** Regular diet.
8. **IV Fluids:** Heparin lock
9. **Special Medications:**

Empiric Therapy for Adults without Gonorrhea Contact:

-Nafcillin or oxacillin 2 gm IV q4h **AND**

Ceftizoxime (Cefizox) 1 gm IV q8h or ceftazidime 1 gm IV q8h or ciprofloxacin 400 mg IV q12h if Gram stain indicates presence of Gram negative organisms.

Empiric Therapy for Adults with Gonorrhea:

-Ceftriaxone (Rocephin) 1 gm IV q12h **OR**

-Ceftizoxime (Cefizox) 1 gm IV q8h **OR**

-Ciprofloxacin (Cipro) 400 mg IV q12h.

-May complete course of therapy with cefuroxime axetil (Ceftin) 400 mg PO bid.

10. **Symptomatic Medications:**

-Acetaminophen and codeine (Tylenol 3) 1-2 PO q4-6h prn pain.

-Heparin 5000 U SQ bid.

11. **Extras:** X-ray views of joint (AP and lateral), CXR. Synovial fluid culture. Physical therapy consult for exercise program.
12. **Labs:** CBC, SMA 7&12, blood C&S x 2, VDRL, UA. Gonorrhea cultures of urethra, cervix, urine, throat, sputum, skin, rectum. Antibiotic levels. Blood cultures x 2 for gonorrhea.

Synovial fluid:

Tube 1 - Glucose, protein, lactate, pH.

Tube 2 - Gram stain, C&S.

Tube 3 - Cell count.

Septic Shock

1. **Admit to:**
2. **Diagnosis:** Sepsis
3. **Condition:**
4. **Vital signs:** q1h; Call physician if BP >160/90, <90/60; P >120, <50; R>25, <10; T >38.5°C; urine output < 25 cc/hr for 4h, O_2 saturation <90%.
5. **Activity:** Bed rest.
6. **Nursing:** Inputs and outputs, pulse oximeter. Foley catheter to closed drainage.
7. **Diet:** NPO
8. **IV Fluids:** 1 liter of normal saline wide open, then D5 ½ NS at 125 cc/h
9. **Special Medications:**

-Oxygen at 2-5 L/min by NC or mask.

Antibiotic Therapy

A. Initial treatment of life-threatening sepsis should include a third-generation cephalosporin (ceftazidime, cefotaxime, ceftizoxime or ceftriaxone), or piperacillin/tazobactam, or ticarcillin/clavulanic acid or imipenem, each with an aminoglycoside (gentamicin, tobramycin or amikacin).

B. **Intra-abdominal or pelvic infections**, likely to involve anaerobes, should be treated with ampicillin, gentamicin and metronidazole; or either ticarcillin/clavulanic acid, ampicillin/sulbactam, piperacillin/tazobactam, imipenem, cefoxitin or cefotetan, each with an aminoglycoside.

C. **Febrile neutropenic patients** with neutrophil counts <500/mm^3 should be treated with vancomycin and ceftazidime, or piperacillin/tazobactam and tobramycin or imipenem and tobramycin.

D. **Dosages for Antibiotics Used in Sepsis**

-Ampicillin 1-2 gm IV q4-6h.
-Cefotaxime (Claforan) 2 gm q4-6h.
-Ceftizoxime (Cefizox) 1-2 gm IV q8h.
-Ceftriaxone (Rocephin) 1-2 gm IV q12h (max 4 gm/d).
-Cefoxitin (Mefoxin) 1-2 gm q6h.
-Cefotetan (Cefotan) 1-2 gm IV q12h.
-Ceftazidime (Fortaz) 1-2 g IV q8h.
-Ticarcillin/clavulanate (Timentin) 3.1 gm IV q4-6h (200-300 mg/kg/d).
-Ampicillin/sulbactam (Unasyn) 1.5-3.0 gm IV q6h.
-Piperacillin/tazobactam (Zosyn) 3.375-4.5 gm IV q6h.
-Piperacillin or ticarcillin 3 gm IV q4-6h.
-Imipenem/cilastatin (Primaxin) 1.0 gm IV q6h.
-Meropenem (Merrem) 05-1.0 gm IV q8h.
-Gentamicin, tobramycin 100-120 mg (1.5 mg/kg) IV, then 80 mg IV q8h (1 mg/kg) or 7 mg/kg in 50 mL of D5W over 60 min IV q24h.
-Amikacin (Amikin) 7.5 mg/kg IV loading dose; then 5 mg/kg IV q8h.
-Vancomycin 1 gm IV q12h.
-Metronidazole (Flagyl) 500 mg (7.5 mg/kg) IV q6-8h.
-Clindamycin 900 mg IV q8h.
-Aztreonam (Azactam) 1-2 gm IV q6-8h; max 8 g/day.

Nosocomial sepsis with IV catheter or IV drug abuse

-Nafcillin or oxacillin 2 gm IV q4h **OR**
-Vancomycin 1 gm q12h (1 gm in 250 cc D5W over 60 min) **AND**
Gentamicin or tobramycin as above **AND EITHER**
Ceftazidime (Fortaz) or ceftizoxime 1-2 gm IV q8h **OR**
Piperacillin, ticarcillin or mezlocillin 3 gm IV q4-6h.

Blood Pressure Support

-Dopamine 4-20 mcg/kg/min (400 mg in 250 cc D5W, 1600 mcg/mL).
-Norepinephrine 2-8 mcg/min IV infusion (8 mg in 250 mL D5W).
-Albumin 25 gm IV (100 mL of 25% sln) **OR**
-Hetastarch (Hespan) 500-1000 cc over 30-60 min (max 1500 cc/d).
-Dobutamine 5 mcg/kg/min, and titrate to bp keep systolic BP >90 mmHg; max 10 mcg/kg/min.

10. Symptomatic Medications:

-Acetaminophen (Tylenol) 650 mg PR q4-6h prn temp >39°C.
-Ranitidine (Zantac) 50 mg IV q8h.
-Heparin 5000 U SQ q12h.

11. Extras: CXR, KUB, ECG. Ultrasound, lumbar puncture.

12. Labs: CBC with differential, SMA 7&12, blood C&S x 3, T&C for 3-6 units PRBC, INR/PTT, drug levels peak and trough at 3rd dose. UA. Cultures of urine, sputum, wound, IV catheters, decubitus ulcers, pleural fluid.

Peritonitis

1. **Admit to:**
2. **Diagnosis:** Peritonitis
3. **Condition:**
4. **Vital signs:** q1-6h. Call physician if BP >160/90, <90/60; P >120, <50; R>25, <10; T >38.5°C.
5. **Activity:** Bed rest.
6. **Nursing:** Guaiac stools.
7. **Diet:** NPO
8. **IV Fluids:** D5 ½ NS at 125 cc/h.
9. **Special Medications:**

Primary Bacterial Peritonitis -- Spontaneous:

Option 1:

-Ampicillin 1-2 gm IV q 4-6h (vancomycin 1 gm IV q12h if penicillin allergic) **AND EITHER**

Cefotaxime (Claforan) 1-2 gm IV q6h **OR**

Ceftizoxime (Cefizox) 1-2 gm IV q8h **OR**

Gentamicin or tobramycin 1.5 mg/kg IV, then 1 mg/kg q8h or 7 mg/kg in 50 mL of D5W over 60 min IV q24h.

Option 2:

-Ticarcillin/clavulanate (Timentin) 3.1 gm IV q6h **OR**

-Piperacillin/tazobactam (Zosyn) 3.375 gm IV q6h **OR**

-Imipenem/cilastatin (Primaxin) 0.5-1.0 gm IV q6h **OR**

-Meropenem (Merrem) 500-1000 mg IV q8h.

Secondary Bacterial Peritonitis -- Abdominal Perforation or Rupture:

Option 1:

-Ampicillin 1-2 gm IV q4-6h **AND**

Gentamicin or tobramycin as above **AND**

Metronidazole (Flagyl) 500 mg IV q8h **OR**

Cefoxitin (Mefoxin) 1-2 gm IV q6h **OR**

Cefotetan (Cefotan) 1-2 gm IV q12h.

Option 2:

-Ticarcillin/clavulanate (Timentin) 3.1 gm IV q4-6h (200-300 mg/kg/d) with an aminoglycoside as above **OR**

-Piperacillin/tazobactam (Zosyn) 3.375 gm IV q6h with an aminoglycoside as above **OR**

-Ampicillin/sulbactam (Unasyn) 1.5-3.0 gm IV q6h with aminoglycoside as above **OR**

-Imipenem/cilastatin (Primaxin) 0.5-1.0 gm IV q6-8h **OR**

-Meropenem (Merrem) 500-1000 mg IV q8h.

Fungal Peritonitis:

-Amphotericin B peritoneal dialysis, 2 mg/L of dialysis fluid over the first 24 hours, then 1.5 mg in each liter **OR**

-Fluconazole (Diflucan) 200 mg IV x 1, then 100 mg IV qd.

10. Symptomatic Medications:

-Ranitidine (Zantac) 50 mg IV q8h.

-Acetaminophen (Tylenol) 325 mg PO/PR q4-6h prn temp >38.5°C.

-Heparin 5000 U SQ q12h.

11. Extras: Plain film, upright abdomen, lateral decubitus, CXR PA and LAT; surgery consult; ECG, abdominal ultrasound. CT scan.

12. Labs: CBC with differential, SMA 7&12, amylase, lactate, INR/PTT, UA with micro, C&S; drug levels peak and trough 3rd dose.

Paracentesis Tube 1: Cell count and differential (1-2 mL, EDTA purple top tube)

Tube 2: Gram stain of sediment; inject 10-20 mL into anaerobic and aerobic culture bottle; AFB, fungal C&S (3-4 mL).

Tube 3: Glucose, protein, albumin, LDH, triglycerides, specific gravity, bilirubin, amylase (2-3 mL, red top tube).

Syringe: pH, lactate (3 mL).

Diverticulitis

1. **Admit to:**
2. **Diagnosis:** Diverticulitis
3. **Condition:**
4. **Vital signs:** qid. Call physician if BP systolic >160/90, <90/60; P >120, <50; R>25, <10; T >38.5°C
5. **Activity:** Up ad lib.
6. **Nursing:** Inputs and outputs.
7. **Diet:** NPO. Advance to clear liquids as tolerated.
8. **IV Fluids:** 0.5-2 L NS over 1-2 hr then, D5 ½ NS at 125 cc/hr. NG tube at low intermittent suction (if obstructed).
9. **Special Medications:**

Regimen 1:

-Gentamicin or tobramycin 100-120 mg IV (1.5-2 mg/kg), then 80 mg IV q8h (5 mg/kg/d) or 7 mg/kg in 50 mL of D5W over 60 min IV q24h **AND EITHER**

Cefoxitin (Mefoxin) 2 gm IV q6-8h **OR**

Clindamycin (Cleocin) 600-900 mg IV q8h.

Regimen 2:

-Metronidazole (Flagyl) 500 mg q8h **AND**

Ciprofloxacin (Cipro) 250-500 mg PO bid or 200-300 mg IV q12h.

Outpatient Regimen:

-Metronidazole (Flagyl) 500 mg PO q6h **AND EITHER**

Ciprofloxacin (Cipro) 500 mg PO bid **OR**

Trimethoprim/SMX (Bactrim) 1 DS tab PO bid.

10. Symptomatic Medications:
-Meperidine (Demerol) 50-100 mg IM or IV q3-4h prn pain.
-Zolpidem (Ambien) 5-10 mg qhs prn insomnia.

11. Extras: Acute abdomen series, CXR PA and LAT, ECG, CT scan of abdomen, ultrasound, surgery and GI consults.

12. Labs: CBC with differential, SMA 7&12, amylase, lipase, blood cultures x 2, drug levels peak and trough 3rd dose. UA, C&S.

Lower Urinary Tract Infection

1. **Admit to:**
2. **Diagnosis:** UTI.
3. **Condition:**
4. **Vital signs:** tid. Call physician if BP <90/60; >160/90; R >30, <10; P >120, <50; T >38.5°C
5. **Activity:** Up ad lib
6. **Nursing:**
7. **Diet:** Regular
8. **IV Fluids:**
9. **Special Medications:**

Lower Urinary Tract Infection (treat for 3-7 days):
-Trimethoprim-sulfamethoxazole (Septra) 1 double strength tab (160/800 mg) PO bid.
-Norfloxacin (Noroxin) 400 mg PO bid.
-Ciprofloxacin (Cipro) 250 mg PO bid.
-Ofloxacin (Floxin) 200 mg PO bid.
-Lomefloxacin (Maxaquin) 400 mg PO qd.
-Enoxacin (Penetrex) 200-400 mg PO q12h; 1h before or 2h after meals.
-Cefpodoxime (Vantin) 100 mg PO bid.
-Cephalexin (Keflex) 500 mg PO q6h.
-Cefixime (Suprax) 200 mg PO q12h or 400 mg PO qd.
-Cefazolin (Ancef) 1-2 gm IV q8h.

Complicated or Catheter-Associated Urinary Tract Infection:
-Ceftizoxime (Cefizox) 1 gm IV q8h.
-Gentamicin 2 mg/kg, then 1.5/kg q8h or 7 mg/kg in 50 mL of D5W over 60 min IV q24h.
-Ticarcillin/clavulanate (Timentin) 3.1 gm IV q4-6h
-Ciprofloxacin (Cipro) 500 mg PO bid.
-Ofloxacin (Floxin) 400 mg PO bid.

Prophylaxis (≥3 episodes/yr):
-Trimethoprim/SMX single strength tab PO qhs.

Candida Cystitis
-Fluconazole (Diflucan) 100 mg PO or IV x 1 dose, then 50 mg PO or IV qd for 5 days **OR**
-Amphotericin B continuous bladder irrigation, 50 mg/1000 mL sterile water via 3-way Foley catheter at 1 L/d for 5 days.

10. Symptomatic Medications:
-Phenazopyridine (Pyridium) 100 mg PO tid.
11. Extras: Renal ultrasound.
12. Labs: CBC, SMA 7. UA with micro, urine Gram stain, C&S.

Pyelonephritis

1. **Admit to:**
2. **Diagnosis:** Pyelonephritis
3. **Condition:**
4. **Vital signs:** tid. Call physician if BP <90/60; >160/90; R >30, <10; P >120, <50; T >38.5°C
5. **Activity:**
6. **Nursing:** Inputs and outputs.
7. **Diet:** Regular
8. **IV Fluids:** D5 ½ NS at 125 cc/h.
9. **Special Medications:**
   -Trimethoprim-sulfamethoxazole (Septra) 160/800 mg (10 mL in 100 mL D5W IV over 2 hours) q12h or 1 double strength tab PO bid.
   -Ciprofloxacin (Cipro) 500 mg PO bid or 400 mg IV q12h.
   -Norfloxacin (Noroxin) 400 mg PO bid
   -Ofloxacin (Floxin) 400 mg PO or IV bid.
   -Levofloxacin (Levaquin) 500 mg PO/IV q24h.
   -In more severely ill patients, treatment with an IV third-generation cephalosporin, or ticarcillin/clavulanic acid, or piperacillin/tazobactam or imipenem is recommended with an aminoglycoside.
   -Ceftizoxime (Cefizox) 1 gm IV q8h.
   -Ceftazidime (Fortaz) 1 gm IV q8h.
   -Ticarcillin/clavulanate (Timentin) 3.1 gm IV q6h.
   -Piperacillin/tazobactam (Zosyn) 3.375 gm IV/PB q6h.
   -Imipenem/cilastatin (Primaxin) 0.5-1.0 gm IV q6-8h.
   -Gentamicin or tobramycin, 2 mg/kg IV, then 1.5 mg/kg q8h or 7 mg/kg in 50 mL of D5W over 60 min IV q24h.
10. **Symptomatic Medications:**
   -Phenazopyridine (Pyridium) 100 mg PO tid.
   -Meperidine (Demerol) 50-100 mg IM q4-6h prn pain.
11. **Extras:** Renal ultrasound, intravenous pyelogram, KUB.
12. **Labs:** CBC with differential, SMA 7. UA with micro, urine Gram stain, C&S; blood C&S x 2. Drug levels peak and trough third dose third dose.

Osteomyelitis

1. **Admit to:**
2. **Diagnosis:** Osteomyelitis
3. **Condition:**
4. **Vital signs:** qid. Call physician if BP <90/60; T >38.5°C
5. **Activity:** Bed rest with bathroom privileges.
6. **Nursing:** Keep involved extremity elevated. Range of motion exercises of upper and lower extremities tid.
7. **Diet:** Regular, high fiber.
8. **IV Fluids:** Heparin lock with flush q shift.
9. **Special Medications:**

Adult Empiric Therapy:

-Nafcillin or oxacillin 2 gm IV q4h **OR**

-Cefazolin (Ancef) 1-2 gm IV q8h **OR**

-Vancomycin 1 gm IV q12h (1 gm in 250 cc D5W over 1h).

-**Add** 3rd generation cephalosporin if gram negative bacilli on Gram stain. Treat for 4-6 weeks.

Post Operative or Post Trauma:

-Vancomycin 1 gm IV q12h **AND** ceftazidime (Fortaz) 1-2 gm IV q8h.

-Imipenem/cilastatin (Primaxin)**(single-drug treatment)** 0.5-1.0 gm IV q6-8h.

-Ticarcillin/clavulanate (Timentin)**(single-drug treatment)** 3.1 gm IV q4-6h.

-Ciprofloxacin (Cipro) 500-750 mg PO bid or 400 mg IV q12h **AND** Rifampin 600 mg PO qd.

Osteomyelitis with Decubitus Ulcer:

-Cefoxitin (Mefoxin), 2 gm IV q6-8h.

-Ciprofloxacin (Cipro) and metronidazole 500 mg IV q8h.

-Imipenem/cilastatin (Primaxin), see dosage above.

-Nafcillin, gentamicin and clindamycin; see dosage above.

10. **Symptomatic Medications:**

-Meperidine (Demerol) 50-100 mg IM q3-4h prn pain.

-Docusate sodium (Colace) 100 mg PO qhs.

-Heparin 5000 U SQ bid.

11. **Extras:** Technetium/gallium bone scans, multiple X-ray views, CT/MRI.
12. **Labs:** CBC with differential, SMA 7, blood C&S x 3, MIC, MBC, UA with micro, C&S. Needle biopsy of bone for C&S; trough antibiotic levels.

Active Pulmonary Tuberculosis

1. **Admit to:**
2. **Diagnosis:** Active Pulmonary Tuberculosis
3. **Condition:**
4. **Vital signs:** q shift
5. **Activity:** Up ad lib in room.
6. **Nursing:** Respiratory isolation.
7. **Diet:** Regular
8. **Special Medications:**
   -Isoniazid 300 mg PO qd (5 mg/kg/d, max 300 mg/d) **AND**
   Rifampin 600 mg PO qd (10 mg/kg/d, 600 mg/d max) **AND**
   Pyrazinamide 500 mg PO bid-tid (15-30 mg/kg/d, max 2.5 gm) **AND**
   Ethambutol 400 mg PO bid-tid (15-25 mg/kg/d, 2.5 gm/d max).
   -Empiric treatment consists of a 4-drug combination of isoniazid (INH), rifampin, pyrazinamide (PZA), and either ethambutol or streptomycin. A modified regimen is recommended for patients known to have INH-resistant TB. Patients are treated for 8 weeks with the four-drug regimen, followed by 18 weeks of INH and rifampin.
   -Pyridoxine 50 mg PO qd with INH.

Prophylaxis
   -Isoniazid 300 mg PO qd (5 mg/kg/d) x 6-9 months.

9. **Extras:** CXR PA, LAT, ECG.
10. **Labs:** CBC with differential, SMA7 and 12, LFTs, HIV serology. First AM sputum for AFB x 3 samples.

Cellulitis

1. **Admit to:**
2. **Diagnosis:** Cellulitis
3. **Condition:**
4. **Vital signs:** tid. Call physician if BP <90/60; T >38.5°C
5. **Activity:** Up ad lib.
6. **Nursing:** Keep affected extremity elevated; warm compresses prn.
7. **Diet:** Regular, encourage fluids.
8. **IV Fluids:** Heparin lock with flush q shift.
9. **Special Medications:**

Empiric Therapy Cellulitis
   -Nafcillin or oxacillin 1-2 gm IV q4-6h **OR**
   -Cefazolin (Ancef) 1-2 gm IV q8h **OR**
   -Vancomycin 1 gm q12h (1 gm in 250 cc D5W over 1h) **OR**
   -Erythromycin 500 IV/PO q6h **OR**
   -Dicloxacillin 500 mg PO qid; may add penicillin VK, 500 mg PO qid, to increase coverage for streptococcus **OR**
   -Cephalexin (Keflex) 500 mg PO qid.

Immunosuppressed, Diabetic Patients, or Ulcerated Lesions:
- -Nafcillin or cefazolin and gentamicin or aztreonam. Add clindamycin or metronidazole if septic.
- -Cefazolin (Ancef) 1-2 gm IV q8h.
- -Cefoxitin (Mefoxin) 1-2 gm IV q6-8h.
- -Gentamicin 2 mg/kg, then 1.5 mg/kg IV q8h or 7 mg/kg in 50 mL of D5W over 60 min IV q24h **OR** aztreonam (Azactam) 1-2 gm IV q6h **PLUS**
- -Metronidazole (Flagyl) 500 mg IV q8h or clindamycin 900 mg IV q8h.
- -Ticarcillin/clavulanate (Timentin) **(single-drug treatment)** 3.1 gm IV q4-6h.
- -Ampicillin/Sulbactam (Unasyn) **(single-drug therapy)** 1.5-3.0 gm IV q6h.
- -Imipenem/cilastatin (Primaxin) **(single-drug therapy)** 0.5-1 mg IV q6-8h.

10. Symptomatic Medications:
- -Acetaminophen/codeine (Tylenol #3) 1-2 PO q4-6h prn pain.

11. Extras: Technetium/Gallium scans, Doppler study (ankle-brachial indices)..

12. Labs: CBC, SMA 7, blood C&S x 2. Leading edge aspirate for Gram stain, C&S; UA, antibiotic levels.

Pelvic Inflammatory Disease

1. **Admit to:**
2. **Diagnosis:** Pelvic Inflammatory Disease
3. **Condition:**
4. **Vital signs:** q8h. Call physician if BP >160/90, <90/60; P >120, <50; R>25, <10; T >38.5°C
5. **Activity:**
6. **Nursing:** Inputs and outputs.
7. **Diet:** Regular
8. **IV Fluids:** D5 ½ NS at 100-125 cc/hr.
9. **Special Medications:**
   - -Cefoxitin (Mefoxin) 2 gm IV q6h **OR** cefotetan (Cefotan) 1-2 gm IV q12h; **AND** doxycycline (Vibramycin) 100 mg IV q12h (IV for 4 days and 48h after afebrile, then complete 10-14 days of doxycycline 100 mg PO bid) **OR**
   - -Clindamycin 900 mg IV q8h **AND** Gentamicin 2 mg/kg IV, then 1.5 mg/kg IV q8h or 7 mg/kg in 50 mL of D5W over 60 min IV q24h, then complete 10-14 d of Clindamycin 300 mg PO qid or Doxycycline 100 mg PO bid **OR**
   - -Ceftriaxone (Rocephin) 250 mg IM x 1 and doxycycline 100 mg PO bid for 14 days **OR**
   - -Ofloxacin (Floxin) 400 mg PO bid for 14 days.

AND EITHER
- -Clindamycin 300 mg PO qid for 14 days **OR**
- -Metronidazole (Flagyl) 500 mg PO bid for 14 days.

10. Symptomatic Medications:
- -Acetaminophen (Tylenol) 1-2 tabs PO q4-6h prn pain or temperature >38.5°C.
- -Meperidine (Demerol) 25-100 mg IM q4-6h prn pain.
- -Zolpidem (Ambien) 10 mg PO qhs prn insomnia.

11. Labs: CBC, SMA 7&12, ESR. GC culture, chlamydia direct fluorescent antibody stain. UA with micro, C&S, VDRL, HIV, blood cultures x 2. Pelvic ultrasound.

Gastrointestinal Disorders

Peptic Ulcer Disease

1. **Admit to:**
2. **Diagnosis:** Peptic ulcer disease.
3. **Condition:**
4. **Vital Signs:** q4h. Call physician if BP >160/90, <90/60; P >120, <50; T >38.5°C
5. **Activity:** Up ad lib
6. **Nursing:** Guaiac stools.
7. **Diet:** NPO 48h, then regular, no caffeine.
8. **IV Fluids:** D5 ½ NS with 20 mEq KCL at 125 cc/h. NG tube at low intermittent suction (if obstructed).
9. **Special Medications:**
   -Ranitidine (Zantac) 50 mg IV bolus, then continuous infusion at 12.5 mg/h (300 mg in 250 mL D5W at 11 mL/h over 24h) or 50 mg IV q8h **OR**
   -Cimetidine (Tagamet) 300 mg IV bolus, then continuous infusion at 50 mg/h (1200 mg in 250 mL D5W over 24h) or 300 mg IV q6-8h **OR**
   -Famotidine (Pepcid) 20 mg IV q12h **OR**
   -Nizatidine (Axid) 300 mg PO qhs **OR**
   -Omeprazole (Prilosec) 20 mg PO bid (30 minutes prior to meals) **OR**
   -Lansoprazole (Prevacid) 15-30 mg PO qd prior to breakfast [15, 30 mg caps].

Eradication of H. pylori

A. **Bismuth, Metronidazole, Tetracycline, Ranitidine**
   1. 14 day therapy.
   2. Bismuth (Pepto bismol) 2 tablets PO qid.
   3. Metronidazole (Flagyl) 250 mg PO qid (tid if cannot tolerate the qid dosing).
   4. Tetracycline 500 mg PO qid.
   5. Ranitidine (Zantac) 150 mg PO bid.
   6. Efficacy is greater than 90%.

B. **Amoxicillin, Omeprazole, Clarithromycin (AOC)**
   1. 10 days of therapy.
   2. Amoxicillin 1 gm PO bid.
   3. Omeprazole (Prilosec) 20 mg PO bid.
   4. Clarithromycin (Biaxin) 500 mg PO bid.

C. **Metronidazole, Omeprazole, Clarithromycin (MOC)**
   1. 10 days of therapy
   2. Metronidazole 500 mg PO bid.
   3. Omeprazole (Prilosec) 20 mg PO bid.
   4. Clarithromycin (Biaxin) 500 mg PO bid.
   5. Efficacy is >80%
   6. Expensive, usually well tolerated.

D. **Omeprazole, Clarithromycin (OC)**
   1. 14 days of therapy.
   2. Omeprazole (Prilosec) 40 mg PO qd for 14 days, then 20 mg qd for an additional 14 days of therapy.
   3. Clarithromycin (Biaxin) 500 mg PO tid.

E. **Ranitidine-Bismuth-Citrate, Clarithromycin (RBC-C)**
   1. 28 days of therapy.
   2. Ranitidine-bismuth-citrate (Tritec) 400 mg PO bid for 28 days.
   3. Clarithromycin 500 mg PO tid for 14 days.
   4. Efficacy is 70-80%; expensive

10. Symptomatic Medications:

-Trimethobenzamide (Tigan) 100-250 mg PO or 100-200 mg IM/PR q6h prn nausea **OR**

-Prochlorperazine (Compazine) 5-10 mg IM/IV/PO q4-6h or 25 mg PR q4-6h prn nausea.

11. Extras: Upright abdomen, KUB, CXR, ECG, endoscopy. GI consult, surgery consult.

12. Labs: CBC, SMA 7&12, amylase, lipase, LDH. UA, Helicobacter pylori serology. Fasting serum gastrin qAM for 3 days. Urea breath test for H pylori.

Gastrointestinal Bleeding

1. **Admit to:**
2. **Diagnosis:** Upper/lower GI bleed
3. **Condition:**
4. **Vital signs:** q30min. Call physician if BP >160/90, <90/60; P >120, <50; R>25, <10; T >38.5°C; urine output <15 mL/hr for 4h.
5. **Activity:** Bed rest
6. **Nursing:** Place nasogastric tube, then lavage with 2 L of room temperature normal saline, then connect to low intermittent suction. Repeat lavage q1h. Record volume and character of lavage. Foley to closed drainage; inputs and outputs.
7. **Diet:** NPO
8. **IV Fluids:** Two 16 gauge IV lines. 1-2 L NS wide open; transfuse 2-6 units PRBC to run as fast as possible, then repeat CBC.
9. **Special Medications:**

-Oxygen 2 L by NC.

-Ranitidine (Zantac) 50 mg IV bolus, then continuous infusion at 12.5 mg/h [300 mg in 250 mL D5W over 24h (11 cc/h)], or 50 mg IV q6-8h **OR**

-Cimetidine (Tagamet) 300 mg IV bolus, then continuous infusion at 50 mg/h (1200 mg in 250 cc D5W over 24h), or 300 mg IV q6-8h **OR**

-Famotidine (Pepcid) 20 mg IV q12h.

-Vitamin K (Phytonadione) 10 mg IV/SQ qd for 3 days (if INR is elevated).

Esophageal Variceal Bleeds:

-Somatostatin (Octreotide) 50 mcg IV bolus, followed by 25-50 mcg/h IV infusion (1200 mcg in 250 mL of D5W at 11 mL/h).

Vasopressin/Nitroglycerine Paste Therapy:

-Vasopressin (Pitressin) 20 U IV over 20-30 minutes, then 0.2-0.3 U/min [100 U in 250 mL of D5W (0.4 U/mL)] for 30 min, followed by increases of 0.2 U/min until bleeding stops or max of 0.9 U/min. If bleeding stops, taper over 24-48h **AND**

-Nitroglycerine paste 1 inch q6h **OR** nitroglycerin IV at 10-30 mcg/min continuous infusion (50 mg in 250 mL of D5W).

10. Extras: Portable CXR, upright abdomen, ECG. Surgery and GI consults.

Upper GI Bleeds: Esophagogastroduodenoscopy with coagulation or sclerotherapy; Linton-Nachlas tube for tamponade of esophageal varices.

Lower GI Bleeds: Sigmoidoscopy/colonoscopy (after a GoLytely purge 6-8 L over 4-6h), technetium 99m RBC scan, angiography with embolization.

11. Labs: Repeat hematocrit q2h; CBC with platelets q12-24h. Repeat INR in 6 hours. SMA 7&12, ALT, AST, alkaline phosphatase, INR/PTT, type and cross for 3-6 U PRBC and 2-4 U FFP.

Cirrhotic Ascites and Edema

1. **Admit to:**
2. **Diagnosis:** Cirrhotic ascites and edema
3. **Condition:**
4. **Vital signs:** Vitals q4-6 hours. Call physician if BP >160/90, <90/60; P >120, <50; T >38.5°C; urine output < 25 cc/hr for 4h.
5. **Activity:** Bed rest with legs elevated.
6. **Nursing:** Inputs and outputs, daily weights, measure abdominal girth qd, guaiac all stools.
7. **Diet:** 2500 calories, 100 gm protein; 500 mg sodium restriction; fluid restriction to 1-1.5 L/d (if hyponatremia, Na <130).
8. **IV Fluids:** Heparin lock with flush q shift.
9. **Special Medications:**

-Diurese to reduce weight by 0.5-1 kg/d (if edema) or 0.25 kg/d (if no edema).

-Spironolactone (Aldactone) 25-50 mg PO qid or 200 mg PO qAM, increase by 100 mg/d to max of 400 mg/d.

-Furosemide (Lasix)(refractory ascites) 40-120 mg PO or IV qd-bid. Add KCL 20-40 mEq PO qAM if renal function is normal **OR**

-Torsemide (Demadex) 20-40 mg PO/IV qd-bid.

-Metolazone (Zaroxolyn) 5-10 mg PO qd (max 20 mg/d).

-Ranitidine (Zantac) 150 mg PO bid.

-Vitamin K 10 mg SQ qd for 3d.

-Folic acid 1 mg PO qd.

-Thiamine 100 mg PO qd.

-Multivitamin PO qd.

Paracentesis: Remove up to 5 L of ascites if peripheral edema, tense ascites, or decreased diaphragmatic excursion. If large volume paracentesis without peripheral edema or with renal insuffiencey, give salt-poor albumin, 12.5 gm for each 2 liters of fluid removed (50 mL of 25%

solution); infuse 25 mL before paracentesis and 25 mL 6h after.

10. Symptomatic Medications:

-Docusate sodium (Colace) 100 mg PO qhs.

-Lactulose 30 mL PO bid-qid.

11. Extras: KUB, CXR, abdominal ultrasound, liver-spleen scan, GI consult.

12. Labs: Ammonia, CBC, SMA 7&12, LFTs, albumin, amylase, lipase, INR/PTT. Urine creatinine, Na, K. HBsAg, anti-HBs, hepatitis C virus antibody, alpha-1-antitrypsin.

Paracentesis Ascitic Fluid

Tube 1: Protein, albumin, specific gravity, glucose, bilirubin, amylase, lipase, triglyceride, LDH (3-5 mL, red top tube).

Tube 2: Cell count and differential (3-5 mL, purple top tube).

Tube 3: C&S, Gram stain, AFB, fungal (5-20 mL); inject 20 mL into blood culture bottles at bedside.

Tube 4: Cytology (>20 mL).

Syringe: pH (2 mL).

Viral Hepatitis

1. **Admit to:**
2. **Diagnosis:** Hepatitis
3. **Condition:**
4. **Vital signs:** qid. Call physician if BP <90/60; T >38.5°C
5. **Activity:**
6. **Nursing:** Stool isolation.
7. **Diet:** Clear liquid (if nausea), low fat (if diarrhea).
8. **Special Medications:**

   -Ranitidine (Zantac) 150 mg PO bid.

   -Vitamin K 10 mg SQ qd for 3d.

   -Multivitamin PO qd.
9. **Symptomatic Medications:**

   -Meperidine (Demerol) 50-100 mg IM q4-6h prn pain.

   -Trimethobenzamide (Tigan) 250 mg PO q6-8h prn pruritus or nausea q6-8h prn.

   -Hydroxyzine (Vistaril) 25 mg IM/PO q4-6h prn pruritus or nausea.

   -Diphenhydramine (Benadryl) 25-50 mg PO/IV q4-6h prn pruritus.
10. **Extras:** Liver/spleen scan, ultrasound, GI consult.
11. **Labs:** CBC, SMA 7&12, GGT, LDH, amylase, lipase, INR/PTT, IgM anti-HAV, IgM anti-HBc, HBsAg, anti-HCV; alpha-1-antitrypsin, ANA, ferritin, ceruloplasmin, urine copper.

Cholecystitis and Cholangitis

1. **Admit to:**
2. **Diagnosis:** Bacterial cholangitis
3. **Condition:**
4. **Vital signs:** q4h. Call physician if BP systolic >160, <90; diastolic. >90, <60; P >120, <50; R>25, <10; T >38.5°C
5. **Activity:** Bed rest
6. **Nursing:** Inputs and outputs
7. **Diet:** NPO
8. **IV Fluids:** 0.5-1 L LR over 1h, then D5 ½ NS with 20 mEq KCL/L at 125 cc/h. NG tube at low constant suction. Foley to closed drainage.
9. **Special Medications:**
   -Ticarcillin or piperacillin 3 gm IV q4-6h, and either metronidazole (Flagyl) 500 mg q8h or cefoxitin (Mefoxin) 1-2 gm IV q6h.
   -Ampicillin 1-2 gm IV q4-6h and gentamicin 100 mg (1.5-2 mg/kg), then 80 mg IV q8h (3-5 mg/kg/d) and metronidazole 500 mg IV q8h.
   -Ticarcillin/clavulanate (Timentin) 3.1 g IV q4-6h (single agent).
   -Imipenem/cilastatin (Primaxin) 1.0 gm IV q6h (single agent).
   -Piperacillin/tazobactam (Zosyn) 3.375 IV q6h.
   -Ampicillin/sulbactam (Unasyn) 1.5-3.0 gm IV q6h.
10. **Symptomatic Medications:**
   -Meperidine (Demerol) 50-100 mg IV/IM q4-6h prn pain.
   -Hydroxyzine (Vistaril) 25-50 mg IV/IM q4-6h prn with meperidine.
   -Omeprazole (Prilosec) 20 mg PO bid.
   -Heparin 5000 U SQ q12h.
11. **Extras:** CXR, ECG, RUQ Ultrasound, HIDA scan, acute abdomen series. GI consult, surgical consult.
12. **Labs:** CBC, SMA 7&12, GGT, amylase, lipase, blood C&S x 2. UA, INR/PTT.

Acute Pancreatitis

1. **Admit to:**
2. **Diagnosis:** Acute pancreatitis
3. **Condition:**
4. **Vital signs:** q1-4h, call physician if BP >160/90, <90/60; P >120, <50; R>25, <10; T >38.5°C; urine output < 25 cc/hr for more than 4 hours.
5. **Activity:** Bed rest with bedside commode.
6. **Nursing:** Inputs and outputs, fingerstick glucose qid, guaiac stools. Foley to closed drainage.
7. **Diet:** NPO
8. **IV Fluids:** 1-4 L NS over 1-3h, then D5 ½ NS with 20 mEq KCL/L at 125 cc/hr. NG tube at low constant suction (if obstruction).

9. Special Medications:

-Ranitidine (Zantac) 12.5 mg/h (300 mg in 250 mL D5W at 11 mL/h) IV or 50 mg IV q6-8h **OR**
Cimetidine (Tagamet) 100 mg/h IV or 300 mg IV q8h **OR**
Famotidine (Pepcid) 20 mg IV q12h.

-Ticarcillin/clavulanate (Timentin) 3.1 gm IV or ampicillin/sulbactam (Unasyn) 3.0 gm IV q6h or imipenem (Primaxin) 0.5-1.0 gm IV q6h.

-Antibiotics are indicated for infected pancreatic pseudocysts or for abscess only. Uncomplicated pancreatitis does not require antibiotics.

-Heparin 5000 U SQ q12h.

-Total parenteral nutrition should be provided until the amylase and lipase are normal and symptoms have resolved.

10. Symptomatic Medications:

-Meperidine 50-100 mg IM/IV q3-4h prn pain.

11. Extras: Upright abdomen, portable CXR, ECG, ultrasound, CT with contrast. Surgery and GI consults.

12. Labs: CBC, platelets, SMA 7&12, calcium, triglycerides, amylase, lipase, LDH, AST, ALT; blood C&S x 2, hepatitis B surface antigen, INR/PTT, type and hold 4-6 U PRBC and 2-4 U FFP. Pancreatic isoamylase, UA.

Acute Diarrhea

1. **Admit to:**
2. **Diagnosis:** Acute Diarrhea
3. **Condition:**
4. **Vital signs:** q6h; call physician if BP >160/90, <80/60; P >120; R>25; T >38.5°C
5. **Activity:** Up ad lib
6. **Nursing:** Daily weights, inputs and outputs.
7. **Diet:** NPO except ice chips for 24h, then low residual elemental diet; no milk products.
8. **IV Fluids:** 1-2 L NS over 1-2 hours; then D5 ½ NS with 40 mEq KCL/L at 125 cc/h.
9. **Special Medications:**

Febrile or gross blood in stool or neutrophils on microscopic exam or prior travel:

-Ciprofloxacin (Cipro) 500 mg PO bid **OR**
-Norfloxacin (Noroxin) 400 mg PO bid **OR**
-Ofloxacin (Floxin) 300 mg bid **OR**
-Trimethoprim/SMX (Bactrim DS) (160/800 mg) one DS tab PO bid.

11. Extras: Upright abdomen. GI consult.

12. Labs: SMA7 and 12, CBC with differential, UA, blood culture x 2.

Stool studies: Wright's stain for fecal leukocytes, ova and parasites x 3, clostridium difficile toxin, culture for enteric pathogens, E coli 0157:H7 culture.

Specific Therapy of Acute Diarrhea

Shigella:
- -Trimethoprim/SMX, (Bactrim) one DS tab PO bid for 5 days **OR**
- -Ciprofloxacin (Cipro) 500 mg PO bid for 5 days **OR**
- -Azithromycin (Zithromax) 500 mg PO x 1, then 250 mg PO qd x 4.

Salmonella (bacteremia):
- -Ofloxacin (Floxin) 400 mg IV/PO q12h for 14 days **OR**
- -Ciprofloxacin (Cipro) 400 mg IV q12h or 750 mg PO q12h for 14 days **OR**
- -Trimethoprim/SMX (Bactrim) one DS tab PO bid for 14 days **OR**
- -Ceftriaxone (Rocephin) 2 gm IV q12h for 14 days.

Campylobacter jejuni:
- -Erythromycin 250 mg PO qid for 5-10 days **OR**
- -Azithromycin (Zithromax) 500 mg PO x 1, then 250 mg PO qd x 4 **OR**
- -Ciprofloxacin (Cipro) 500 mg PO bid for 5 days.

Enterotoxic/Enteroinvasive E coli (Travelers Diarrhea):
- -Ciprofloxacin (Cipro) 500 mg PO bid for 5-7 days **OR**
- -Trimethoprim/SMX (Bactrim), one DS tab PO bid for 5-7 days.

Antibiotic-Associated and Pseudomembranous Colitis (Clostridium difficile):
- -Metronidazole (Flagyl) 250 mg PO or IV qid for 10-14 days **OR**
- -Vancomycin 125 mg PO qid for 10 days (500 PO qid for 10-14 days, if recurrent).

Yersinia Enterocolitica (sepsis):
- -Trimethoprim/SMX (Bactrim), one DS tab PO bid for 5-7 days **OR**
- -Ciprofloxacin (Cipro) 500 mg PO bid for 5-7 days **OR**
- -Ofloxacin (Floxin) 400 mg PO bid **OR**
- -Ceftriaxone (Rocephin) 1 gm IV q12h.

Entamoeba Histolytica (Amebiasis):

Mild to Moderate Intestinal Disease:
- -Metronidazole (Flagyl) 750 mg PO tid for 10 days **OR**
- -Tinidazole 2 gm per day PO for 3 days **Followed By:**
- -Iodoquinol 650 mg PO tid for 20 days **OR**
- -Paromomycin 25-30 mg/kg/d PO tid for 7 days.

Severe Intestinal Disease:
- -Metronidazole (Flagyl)750 mg PO tid for 10 days **OR**
- -Tinidazole 600 mg PO bid for 5 days **Followed By:**
- -Iodoquinol 650 mg PO tid for 20 days **OR**
- -Paromomycin 25-30 mg/kg/d PO tid for 7 days.

Giardia Lamblia:
- -Quinacrine 100 mg PO tid for 5d **OR**
- -Metronidazole 250 mg PO tid for 7 days.

Cryptosporidium:
- -Paromomycin 500 mg PO qid for 7-10 days [250 mg].

Crohn's Disease

1. **Admit to:**
2. **Diagnosis:** Crohn's disease.
3. **Condition:**
4. **Vital signs:** q8h. Call physician if BP >160/90, <90/60; P >120, <50; R>25, <10; T >38.5°C
5. **Activity:** Up ad lib in room.
6. **Nursing:** Inputs and outputs. NG at low intermittent suction (if obstruction).
7. **Diet:** NPO except for ice chips and medications for 48h, then low residue or elemental diet, no milk products.
8. **IV Fluids:** 1-2 L NS over 1-3h, then D5 ½ NS with 40 mEq KCL/L at 125 cc/hr.
9. **Special Medications:**
   - -Mesalamine (Asacol) 400-800 mg PO tid or mesalamine (Pentasa) 1000 mg (four 250 mg tabs) PO qid **OR**
   - -Sulfasalazine (Azulfidine) 0.5-1 gm PO bid; increase over 10 days to 0.5-1 gm PO qid **OR**
   - -Olsalazine (Dipentum) 500 mg PO bid.
   - -Infliximab (Remicade) 5 mg/kg IV over 2 hours; MR at 2 and 6 weeks
   - -Prednisone 40-60 mg/d PO in divided doses **OR**
   - -Hydrocortisone 50-100 mg IV q6h **OR**
   - -Methylprednisolone (Solu-Medrol) 10-20 mg IV q6h.
   - -Metronidazole (Flagyl) 250-500 mg PO q6h.
   - -Vitamin B_{12}, 100 mcg IM for 5d then 100-200 mcg IM q month.
   - -Multivitamin PO qAM or 1 ampule IV qAM.
   - -Folic acid 1 mg PO qd.
10. **Extras:** Abdominal x-ray series, CXR. GI consult.
11. **Labs:** CBC, SMA 7&12, Mg, ionized calcium, blood C&S x 2; stool Wright's stain, stool culture, C difficile antigen assay, stool ova and parasites x 3.

Ulcerative Colitis

1. **Admit to:**
2. **Diagnosis:** Ulcerative colitis
3. **Condition:**
4. **Vital signs:** q4-6h. Call physician if BP >160/90, <90/60; P >120, <50; R>25, <10; T >38.5°C
5. **Activity:** Up ad lib in room.
6. **Nursing:** Inputs and outputs.
7. **Diet:** NPO except for ice chips for 48h, then low residue or elemental diet, no milk products.
8. **IV Fluids:** 1-2 L NS over 1-2h, then D5 ½ NS with 40 mEq KCL/L at 125 cc/hr.

9. **Special Medications:**
   - -Mesalamine (Asacol) 400-800 mg PO tid **OR**
   - -5-aminosalicylate (Mesalamine) 400-800 mg PO tid or 1 gm PO qid or enema 4 gm/60 mL PR qhs **OR**
   - -Sulfasalazine (Azulfidine) 0.5-1 gm PO bid, increase over 10 days as tolerated to 0.5-1.0 gm PO qid **OR**
   - -Olsalazine (Dipentum) 500 mg PO bid **OR**
   - -Hydrocortisone retention enema, 100 mg in 120 mL saline bid.
   - -Methylprednisolone (Solu-Medrol) 10-20 mg IV q6h **OR**
   - -Hydrocortisone 100 mg IV q6h **OR**
   - -Prednisone 40-60 mg/d PO in divided doses.
   - -B12, 100 mcg IM for 5d then 100-200 mcg IM q month.
   - -Multivitamin,PO qAM or 1 ampule IV qAM.
   - -Folate 1 mg PO qd.
10. **Symptomatic Medications:**
    - -Loperamide (Imodium) 2-4 mg PO tid-qid prn, max 16 mg/d **OR**
    - -Kaopectate 60-90 mL PO qid prn.
11. **Extras:** Upright abdomen. CXR, colonoscopy, GI consult.
12. **Labs:** CBC, SMA 7&12, Mg, ionized calcium, liver panel, blood C&S x 2; stool Wright's stain, stool for ova and parasites x 3, culture for enteric pathogens; Clostridium difficile antigen assay, UA.

Parenteral Nutrition

General Considerations: Daily weights, inputs and outputs. Finger stick glucose q6h.

Central Parenteral Nutrition:

- -Infuse 40-50 mL/h of amino acid-dextrose solution in the first 24h; increase daily by 40 mL/hr increments until providing 1.3-2 x basal energy requirement and 1.2-1.7 gm protein/kg/d (see formula page 97).

Standard solution:

Amino acid sln (Aminosyn) 7-10%	500 mL
Dextrose 40-70%	500 mL
Sodium	35 mEq
Potassium	36 mEq
Chloride	35 mEq
Calcium	4.5 mEq
Phosphate	9 mmol
Magnesium	8.0 mEq
Acetate	82-104 mEq
Multi-trace element formula (Zn, copper, manganese, chromium)	1 mL/d
Regular insulin (if indicated)	10-60 U/L
Multivitamin(12)(2 amp)	10 mL/d
Vitamin K (in solution, SQ, IM)	10 mg/week
Vitamin B12	1000 mcg/week

Selenium (after 20 days of continuous TPN) . . . . 80 mcg/d

Intralipid 20%, 500 mL/d IVPB; infuse in parallel with standard solution at 1 mL/min for 15 min; if no adverse reactions, increase to 100 mL/hr once daily or 20 mg/hr continuously. Obtain serum triglyceride 6h after end of infusion (maintain <250 mg/dL).

Cyclic Total Parenteral Nutrition:

-12h night schedule; taper continuous infusion in morning by reducing rate to half of original rate for 1 hour. Further reduce rate by half for an additional hour, then discontinue. Finger stick glucose q4-6h; restart TPN in afternoon. Taper at beginning and end of cycle. Final rate of 185 mL/hr for 9-10 h and 2 hours of taper at each end for total of 2000 mL.

Peripheral Parenteral Supplementation:

-3% amino acid sln (ProCalamine) up to 3 L/d at 125 cc/h **OR**

-Combine 500 mL amino acid solution 7% or 10% (Aminosyn) and 500 mL 20% dextrose and electrolyte additive. Infuse at up to 100 cc/hr in parallel with:

-Intralipid 10% or 20% at 1 mL/min for 15 min (test dose); if no adverse reactions, infuse 500 mL/d at 21 mL/h over 24h, or up to 100 mL/h over 5 hours daily.

-Draw triglyceride level 6h after end of Intralipid infusion.

7. **Special Medications:**
   -Cimetidine (Tagamet) 300 mg IV q6-8h or 1200 mg/day in TPN **OR**
   -Ranitidine (Zantac) 50 mg IV q8h or 150 mg/day in TPN.
8. **Extras:** Nutrition consult.
9. **Labs:**
   Daily labs: SMA7, osmolality, CBC, cholesterol, triglyceride, urine glucose and specific gravity.
   Twice weekly Labs: Calcium, phosphate, SMA-12, magnesium
   Weekly Labs: Serum albumin and protein, pre-albumin, ferritin, INR/PTT, zinc, copper, B12, folate, 24h urine nitrogen and creatinine.

Enteral Nutrition

General Considerations: Daily weights, inputs and outputs, nasoduodenal feeding tube. Head-of-bed at 30° while enteral feeding and 2 hours after completion.

Enteral Bolus Feeding: Give 50-100 mL of enteral solution (Pulmocare, Jevity, Vivonex, Osmolite, Vital HN) q3h. Increase amount in 50 mL steps to max of 250-300 mL q3-4h; 30 kcal of nonprotein calories/kg/d and 1.5 gm protein/kg/d. Before each feeding measure residual volume, and delay feeding by 1h if >100 mL. Flush tube with 100 cc of water after each bolus.

Continuous enteral infusion: Initial enteral solution (Pulmocare, Jevity, Vivonex, Osmolite) 30 mL/hr. Measure residual volume q1h for 12h then tid; hold feeding for 1h if >100 mL. Increase rate by 25-50 mL/hr at 24 hr intervals as tolerated until final rate of 50-100 mL/hr. Three tablespoonfuls of protein powder (Promix) may be added to each 500 cc of solution. Flush tube with 100 cc water q8h.

Special Medications:

-Metoclopramide (Reglan) 10-20 mg PO or in J-tube q6h **OR**

-Cisapride (Propulsid) 10-20 mg via nasogastric tube qid (concurrent use with macrolide antibiotics or azole antifungals may result in prolongation of QT interval) **OR**

-Erythromycin 125 mg IV or via nasogastric tube q8h.

-Cimetidine (Tagamet) 400 mg PO bid **OR**

-Ranitidine (Zantac)150 mg PO bid.

Symptomatic Medications:

-Loperamide (Imodium) 2-4 mg PO/J-tube q6h prn, max 16 mg/d **OR**

-Diphenoxylate/atropine (Lomotil) 1-2 tabs or 5-10 mL (2.5 mg/5 mL) PO/J-tube q4-6h prn, max 12 tabs/d **OR**

-Kaopectate 30 cc PO or in J-tube q8h.

Extras: CXR, plain abdominal x-ray for tube placement, nutrition consult.

Labs:

Daily labs: SMA7, osmolality, CBC, cholesterol, triglyceride. SMA-12

Weekly Labs when indicated: Protein, Mg, INR/PTT, 24h urine nitrogen and creatinine. Pre-albumin, retinol-binding protein.

Hepatic Encephalopathy

1. **Admit to:**
2. **Diagnosis:** Hepatic encephalopathy
3. **Condition:**
4. **Vital signs:** q1-4h, neurochecks q4h. Call physician if BP >160/90,<90/60; P >120,<50; R>25,<10; T >38.5°C
5. **Allergies:** Avoid sedatives, NSAIDS or hepatotoxic drugs.
6. **Activity:** Bed rest.
7. **Nursing:** Keep head-of-bed at 40 degrees, guaiac stools; turn patient q2h while awake, chart stools. Seizure precautions, egg crate mattress, soft restraints prn. Record inputs and outputs.
8. **Diet:** Low protein nasogastric enteral feedings (Hepatic-Aid II) at 30 mL/hr. Increase rate by 25-50 mL/hr at 24 hr intervals as tolerated until final rate of 50-100 mL/hr as tolerated. No dietary protein for 8 hours.
9. **IV Fluids:** D5W at TKO, Foley to closed drainage.
10. **Special Medications:**

-Sorbitol 500 mL in 200 mL of water PO now.

-Lactulose 30-45 mL PO q1h for 3 doses, then 15-45 mL PO bid-qid, titrate to produce 3 soft stools/d **OR**

-Lactulose enema 300 mL in 700 mL of tap water; instill 200-250 mL per rectal tube bid-qid. **AND**

-Neomycin 1 gm PO q4-6h (4-12 g/d) **OR**

-Metronidazole (Flagyl) 250 mg PO q6h.

-Ranitidine (Zantac) 50 mg IV q8h or 150 mg PO bid **OR**

-Famotidine (Pepcid) 20 mg IV/PO q12h.

-Flumazenil (Romazicon) 0.2 mg (2 mL) IV over 30 seconds q1min until a total dose of 3 mg; if a partial response occurs, continue 0.5 mg doses until a total of 5 mg. Flumazenil may help reverse hepatic encephalopathy, even in the absence of benzodiazepine use. Excessive doses of flumazenil may precipitate seizures.

-Multivitamin PO qAM or 1 ampule IV qAM.

-Folic acid 1 mg PO/IV qd.

-Thiamine 100 mg PO/IV qd.

-Vitamin K 10 mg SQ qd for 3 days if elevated INR.

11. Extras: CXR, ECG; GI and dietetics consults.

12. Labs: Ammonia, CBC, platelets, SMA 7&12, AST, ALT, GGT, LDH, alkaline phosphatase, protein, albumin, bilirubin, INR/PTT, ABG, blood C&S x 2, hepatitis B surface antibody. UA.

Alcohol Withdrawal

1. **Admit to:**
2. **Diagnosis:** Alcohol withdrawals/delirium tremens.
3. **Condition:**
4. **Vital signs:** q4-6h. Call physician if BP >160/90, <90/60; P >130, <50; R>25, <10; T >38.5°C; or increase in agitation.
5. **Activity:**
6. **Nursing:** Seizure precautions. Soft restraints prn.
7. **Diet:** Regular, push fluids.
8. **IV Fluids:** Heparin lock or D5 ½ NS at 100-125 cc/h.
9. **Special Medications:**

Withdrawal syndrome:

-Chlordiazepoxide (Librium) 50-100 mg PO/IV q6h for 3 days.

Delirium tremens:

-Chlordiazepoxide (Librium) 100 mg slow IV push or PO, repeat q4-6h prn agitation or tremor for 24h; max 500 mg/d. Then give 50-100 mg PO q6h prn agitation or tremor **OR**

-Diazepam (Valium) 5 mg slow IV push, repeat q6h until calm, then 5-10 mg PO q4-6h.

-Magnesium sulfate 1-8 gm in 100 mL D5W IV over 2h qd.

Seizures:

-Thiamine 100 mg IV push **AND**

-Dextrose water 50%, 50 mg IV push.

-Lorazepam (Ativan) 0.1 mg/kg IV at 2 mg/min; may repeat x 1 if seizures continue.

Wernicke-Korsakoff Syndrome:

-Thiamine 100 mg IV stat, then 100 mg IV qd.

10. Symptomatic Medications:

-Multivitamin 1 amp IV, then 1 tab PO qd.

-Folate 1 mg PO qd.

-Thiamine 100 mg PO qd.
-Acetaminophen (Tylenol) 1-2 PO q4-6h prn headache.

11. Extras: CXR, ECG. Alcohol rehabilitation and social work consult.

12. Labs: CBC, SMA 7&12, Mg, amylase, lipase, liver panel, urine drug screen. UA, INR/PTT.

Toxicology

Poisoning and Drug Overdose

Decontamination:

-Gastric Lavage: Place patient left side down, place nasogastric tube, and check position by injecting air and auscultating. Lavage with normal saline until clear fluid, then leave activated charcoal or other antidote. Gastric lavage is contraindicated for corrosives.

-Cathartics:

-Magnesium citrate 6% sln 150-300 mL PO

-Magnesium sulfate 10% solution 150-300 mL PO.

-Activated Charcoal: 50 gm PO (first dose should be given using product containing sorbitol). Repeat q2-6h for large ingestions.

-Hemodialysis: Indicated for isopropanol, methanol, ethylene glycol, severe salicylate intoxication (>100 mg/dL), lithium, or theophylline (if neurotoxicity, seizures, or coma).

Antidotes:

Narcotic Overdose:

-Naloxone (Narcan) 0.4 mg IV/ET/IM/SC, may repeat q2min.

Methanol Ingestion:

-Ethanol (10% in D5W) 7.5 mL/kg load, then 1.4 mL/kg/hr IV infusion until methanol level <20 mg/dL. Maintain ethanol level of 100-150 mg/100 mL.

Ethylene Glycol Ingestion:

-Fomepizole (Antizol) 15 mg/kg IV over 30 min, then 10 mg/kg IV q12h x 4 doses, then 15 mg/kg IV q12h until ethylene glycol level is less than 20 mg/dL **AND**

-Pyridoxine 100 mg IV q6h for 2 days and thiamine 100 mg IV q6h for 2 days

Carbon Monoxide Intoxication:

-Hyperbaric oxygen therapy or 100% oxygen by mask if hyperbaric oxygen not available.

Tricyclic Antidepressants Overdose:

-Gastric lavage

-Magnesium citrate 300 mg PO/NG x1

-Activated charcoal premixed with sorbitol 50 gm NG q4-6h until level is less than the toxic range.

Benzodiazepine Overdose:

-Flumazenil (Romazicon) 0.2 mg (2 mL) IV over 30 seconds q1min until a total dose of 3 mg; if a partial response occurs, repeat 0.5 mg doses until a total of 5 mg. If sedation persists, repeat the above regimen or start a continuous IV infusion of 0.1-0.5 mg/h. Excessive doses may cause seizures.

Labs: Drug screen (serum, gastric, urine); blood levels, SMA 7, fingerstick glucose, CBC, LFTs, ECG.

Acetaminophen Overdose

1. **Admit to:** Medical intensive care unit.
2. **Diagnosis:** Acetaminophen overdose
3. **Condition:**
4. **Vital signs:** q1h with neurochecks. Call physician if BP >160/90, <90/60; P >130, <50 <50; R>25, <10; urine output <20 cc/h for 3 hours.
5. **Activity:** Bed rest with bedside commode.
6. **Nursing:** Inputs and outputs, aspiration and seizure precautions. Place large bore (Ewald) NG tube, then lavage with 2 L of NS.
7. **Diet:** NPO
8. **IV Fluids:**
9. **Special Medications:**
   - -Activated Charcoal 30-100 gm doses, remove via NG suction prior to acetylcysteine.
   - -Acetylcysteine (Mucomyst, NAC) 5% solution loading dose 140 mg/kg via NG tube, then 70 mg/kg via NG tube q4h x 17 doses **OR** acetylcysteine 150 mg/kg IV in 200 mL D5W over 15 min, followed by 50 mg/kg in 500 mL D5W, infused over 4h, followed by 100 mg/kg in 1000 mL of D5W over next 16h. Complete all NAC doses even if acetaminophen levels fall below toxic range.
   - -Phytonadione 5 mg IV/IM/SQ (if INR increased).
   - -Fresh frozen plasma 2-4 U (if INR is unresponsive to phytonadione).
   - -Trimethobenzamide (Tigan) 100-200 mg IM/PR q6h prn nausea
10. **Extras:** ECG. Nephrology consult for hemodialysis or charcoal hemoperfusion.
11. **Labs:** CBC, SMA 7&12, LFTs, INR/PTT, acetaminophen level now and in 4h. UA.

Theophylline Overdose

1. **Admit to:** Medical intensive care unit.
2. **Diagnosis:** Theophylline overdose
3. **Condition:**
4. **Vital signs:** Neurochecks q2h. Call physician if BP >160/90, <90/60; P >130; <50; R >25, <10.
5. **Activity:** Bed rest
6. **Nursing:** ECG monitoring until level <20 mcg/mL, aspiration and seizure precautions. Insert single lumen NG tube and lavage with normal saline if recent ingestion.
7. **Diet:** NPO
8. **IV Fluids:** D5 ½ NS at 125 cc/h

9. **Special Medications:**
   - -Activated charcoal 50 gm PO q4-6h, with sorbitol cathartic, until theophylline level <20 mcg/mL. Maintain head-of-bed at 30-45 degrees to prevent aspiration of charcoal.
   - -Charcoal hemoperfusion is indicated if the serum level is >60 mcg/mL or if signs of neurotoxicity, seizure, coma are present.
   - -**Seizure:** Lorazepam 0.1 mg/kg IV at 2 mg/min; may repeat x 1 if seizures continue.
10. **Extras:** ECG.
11. **Labs:** CBC, SMA 7&12, theophylline level now and in q6-8h; INR/PTT, liver panel. UA.

Tricyclic Antidepressant Overdose

1. **Admit to:** Medical intensive care unit.
2. **Diagnosis:** TCA Overdose
3. **Condition:**
4. **Vital Signs:** Neurochecks q1h.
5. **Activity:** Bedrest.
6. **Nursing:** Continuous suicide observation. ECG monitoring, measure QRS width hourly, inputs and outputs, aspiration and seizure precautions. Place single-lumen nasogastric tube and lavage with 2 liters of normal saline if recent ingestion.
7. **Diet:** NPO
8. **IV Fluids:** NS at 100-150 cc/hr.
9. **Special Medications:**
   - -Activated charcoal premixed with sorbitol 50 gm via NG tube q4-6h until the TCA level decreases to therapeutic range. Maintain head-of-bed at 30-45 degree angle to prevent charcoal aspiration.
   - -Magnesium citrate 300 mL via nasogastric tube x 1 dose.
10. **Cardiac Toxicity:**
    - -If mechanical ventilation is necessary, hyperventilate to maintain pH 7.50-7.55.
    - -Administer sodium bicarbonate 50-100 mEq (1-2 amps or 1-2 mEq/kg) IV over 5-10 min, followed by infusion of sodium bicarbonate (2 amps in D5W 1 L) at 100-150 cc/h. Adjust rate to maintain pH 7.50-7.55.
11. **Extras:** ECG.
12. **Labs:** Urine toxicology screen, serum TCA levels, liver panel, CBC, SMA-7 and 12, UA.

Neurologic Disorders

Ischemic Stroke

1. **Admit to:**
2. **Diagnosis:** Ischemic stroke
3. **Condition:**
4. **Vital signs:** Vital signs and neurochecks q30minutes for 6 hours, then q60 minutes for 12 hours. Call physician if BP >185/105, <110/60; P >120, <50; R>24, <10; T >38.5°C; or change in neurologic status.
5. **Activity:** Bedrest.
6. **Nursing:** Head-of-bed at 30 degrees, turn q2h when awake, range of motion exercises qid. Foley catheter, eggcrate mattress. Guaiac stools, inputs and outputs's. Oxygen at 2 L per minute by nasal cannula.
   Bleeding precautions: check puncture sites for bleeding or hematomas. Apply digital pressure or pressure dressing to active compressible bleeding sites.
7. **Diet:** NPO except medications for 24 hours, then dysphagia ground diet with thickened liquids.
8. **IV Fluids:** 0.45% normal saline at 100 cc/h.
9. **Special Medications:**

Ischemic Stroke < 3 hours:

-Tissue plasminogen activator (t-PA, Alteplase) is indicated if the patient presents within 3 hours of onset of symptoms and the stroke is non-hemorrhagic; 0.9 mg/kg (max 90 mg) over 60 min, with 10% of the total dose given as an initial bolus over 1 minute.

Completed Ischemic Stroke >3 hours:

-Aspirin enteric coated 325 mg PO qd **OR**
-Clopidogrel (Plavix) 75 mg PO qd **OR**
-Ticlopidine (Ticlid) 250 mg PO bid.

10. **Symptomatic Medications:**

-Ranitidine (Zantac) 50 mg IV q8h or 150 mg PO bid
-Omeprazole (Prilosec) 20 mg PO bid or qhs.
-Docusate sodium (Colace) 100 mg PO qhs
-Bisacodyl (Dulcolax) 10-15 mg PO qhs or 10 mg PR prn.
-Acetaminophen (Tylenol) 650 mg PO/PR q4-6h prn temp >38°C or headache.

11. **Extras:** CXR, ECG, CT without contrast or MRI with gadolinium contrast; carotid duplex scan; echocardiogram, 24-hour Holter monitor; swallowing studies. Physical therapy consult for range of motion exercises; neurology, rehabilitation medicine consults.

12. **Labs:** CBC, glucose, SMA 7&12, fasting lipid profile, VDRL, ESR; drug levels, INR/PTT, UA. Lupus anticoagulant, anticardiolipin antibody.

Transient Ischemic Attack

1. **Admit to:**
2. **Diagnosis:** Transient ischemic attack
3. **Condition:**
4. **Vital signs:** q1h with neurochecks. Call physician if BP >160/90, <90/60; P >120, <50; R>25, <10; T >38.5°C; or change in neurologic status.
5. **Activity:** Up as tolerated.
6. **Nursing:** Guaiac stools.
7. **Diet:** Dysphagia ground with thickened liquids or regular diet.
8. **IV Fluids:** Heparin lock with flush q shift.
9. **Special Medications:**
   -Aspirin 325 mg PO qd **OR**
   -Clopidogrel (Plavix) 75 mg PO qd **OR**
   -Ticlopidine (Ticlid) 250 mg PO bid **OR**
   -Heparin (only if recurrent TIAs or cardiogenic or vertebrobasilar source for emboli) 700-800 U/h (12 U/kg/h) IV infusion without a bolus (25,000 U in 500 mL D5W); adjust q6-12h until PTT 1.2-1.5 x control.
   -Warfarin (Coumadin) 5.0-7.5 mg PO qd for 3d, then 2-4 mg PO qd. Titrate to INR of 2.0-2.5.
10. **Symptomatic Medications:**
   -Ranitidine (Zantac) 150 mg PO bid.
   -Docusate sodium (Colace) 100 mg PO qhs.
   -Milk of magnesia 30 mL PO qd prn constipation.
11. **Extras:** CXR, ECG, CT without contrast; carotid duplex scan, echocardiogram, 24-hour Holter monitor. Physical therapy, neurology consults.
12. **Labs:** CBC, glucose, SMA 7&12, fasting lipid profile, VDRL, drug levels, INR/PTT, UA.

Subarachnoid Hemorrhage

Treatment:

-Stat neurosurgery consult.

-Head of bed at 20 degrees, turn patient q2h, range of motion exercises qid, Foley catheter, eggcrate mattress. Guaiac stools.

-Keep room dark and quiet; strict bedrest. Neurologic checks q1h for 12 hours, then q2h for 12 hours, then q4h. Call physician if abrupt change in neurologic status.

-Restrict total fluids to 1000 mL/day; diet as tolerated.

-Nimodipine (Nimotop) 60 mg PO or via NG tube q4h for 21d, must start within 96 hours.

-Phenytoin (seizures) load 15 mg/kg IV in NS (infuse at max 50 mg/min), then 300 mg PO/IV qAM (4-6 mg/kg/d).

Hypertension:

-Nitroprusside sodium, 0.1-0.5 mcg/kg/min (50 mg in 250 mL NS), titrate to control blood pressure.

Extras: CXR, ECG, CT without contrast; MRI angiogram; cerebral angiogram. Neurology, neurosurgery consults.
Labs: CBC, SMA 7&12, VDRL, UA.

Seizure and Status Epilepticus

1. **Admit to:**
2. **Diagnosis:** Seizure
3. **Condition:**
4. **Vital signs:** q1h with neurochecks. Call physician if BP >160/90, <90/60; P >120, <50; R>25, <10; T >38.5°C; or any change in neurological status.
5. **Activity:** Bed rest
6. **Nursing:** Finger stick glucose. Seizure precautions with bed rails up; padded tongue blade at bedside. EEG monitoring.
7. **Diet:** NPO for 24h, then regular diet if alert.
8. **IV Fluids:** D5 ½ NS at 100 cc/hr; change to heparin lock when taking PO.
9. **Special Medications:**

Status Epilepticus:

1. Maintain airway.
2. Position the patient laterally with the head down. The head and extremities should be cushioned to prevent injury.
3. During the tonic portion of the seizure, the teeth are tightly clenched. During the clonic phase that follows, however, a bite block or other soft object should be inserted into the mouth to prevent injury to the tongue.
4. 100% O_2 by mask, obtain brief history, and a fingerstick glucose.
5. Secure IV access and draw blood for serum glucose analysis. Give thiamine 100 mg IV push to prevent Wernicke's encephalopathy, then dextrose 50% 50 mL IV push.
6. **Initial Control:**
   - **Lorazepam (Ativan)** 6-8 mg (0.1 mg/kg; not to exceed 2 mg/min) IV at 1-2 mg/min. May repeat 6-8 mg q5-10min (max 80 mg/24h) **OR**
   - **Diazepam (Valium)**, 5-10 mg slow IV at 1-2 mg/min. Repeat 5-10 mg q5-10 min prn (max 100 mg/24h).
   - **Phenytoin (Dilantin)** 15-20 mg/kg load in NS at 50 mg/min. Repeat 100-150 mg IV q30min, max 1.5 gm; monitor BP.
   - **Fosphenytoin (Cerebyx)** 20 mg/kg IV/IM (at 150 mg/min), then 4-6 mg/kg/day in 2 or 3 doses (150 mg IV/IM q8h). Fosphenytoin is metabolized to phenytoin; fosphenytoin may be given IM.
   - **If Seizures Persist, Administer Phenobarbital** 20 mg/kg IV at 50 mg/min, repeat 2 mg/kg q15min; additional phenobarbital may be given, up to max of 30-60 mg/kg.
7. **If Seizures Persist, Intubate the Patient and Consider:**
   - Midazolam (Versed) 0.2 mg/kg IV push, then 0.045 mg/kg/hr; titrate up to 0.6 mg/kg/hr **OR**
   - Propofol (Diprivan) 2 mg/kg IV push, then 2 mg/kg/hr; titrate up to 10 mg/kg/hr **OR**

-Phenobarbital as above.
-Induction of coma with pentobarbital 10-15 mg/kg IV over 1-2h, then 1-1.5 mg/kg/h continuous infusion. Initiate continuous EEG monitoring.

8. **Consider Intubation and General Anesthesia**

Maintenance Therapy for Epilepsy:

Primary Generalized Seizures -- First-Line Therapy:

-Carbamazepine (Tegretol) 200-400 mg PO tid [100, 200 mg]. Monitor CBC.
-Phenytoin (Dilantin) loading dose of 400 mg PO followed by 300 mg PO q4h for 2 doses (total of 1 g), then 300 mg PO qd or 100 mg tid or 200 mg bid [30, 50, 100 mg].
-Divalproex (Depakote) 250-500 mg PO tid-qid with meals [125, 250, 500 mg].
-Valproic acid (Depakene) 250-500 mg PO tid-qid with meals [250 mg].

Primary Generalized Seizures -- Second Line Therapy:

-Phenobarbital 30-120 mg PO bid [8, 16, 32, 65, 100 mg].
-Primidone (Mysoline) 250-500 mg PO tid [50, 250 mg]; metabolized to phenobarbital.
-Felbamate (Felbatol) 1200-2400 mg PO qd in 3-4 divided doses, max 3600 mg/d [400, 600 mg; 600 mg/5 mL susp]; adjunct therapy; aplastic anemia, hepatotoxicity.
-Gabapentin (Neurontin), 300-400 mg PO bid-tid; max 1800 mg/day [100, 300, 400 mg]; adjunct therapy.
-Lamotrigine (Lamictal) 50 mg PO qd, then increase to 50-250 mg PO bid [25, 100, 150, 200 mg]; adjunct therapy .

Partial Seizure:

-Carbamazepine (Tegretol) 200-400 mg PO tid [100, 200 mg].
-Divalproex (Depakote) 250-500 mg PO tid with meals [125, 250, 500 mg].
-Valproic acid (Depakene) 250-500 mg PO tid-qid with meals [250 mg].
-Phenytoin (Dilantin) 300 mg PO qd or 200 mg PO bid [30, 50, 100].
-Phenobarbital 30-120 mg PO tid or qd [8, 16, 32, 65, 100 mg].
-Primidone (Mysoline) 250-500 mg PO tid [50, 250 mg]; metabolized to phenobarbital.
-Felbamate (Felbatol) 1200-2400 mg PO qd in 3-4 divided doses, max 3600 mg/d [400,600 mg; 600 mg/5 mL susp]; adjunct therapy; aplastic anemia, hepatotoxicity.
-Gabapentin (Neurontin), 300-400 mg PO bid-tid; max 1800 mg/day [100, 300, 400 mg]; adjunct therapy.
-Lamotrigine (Lamictal) 50 mg PO qd, then increase to 50-250 mg PO bid [25, 100, 150, 200 mg]; adjunct therapy.
-Topiramate (Topamax) 25 mg PO bid; titrate to max 200 mg PO bid [tab 25, 100, 200 mg]; adjunctive therapy.

Absence Seizure:

-Divalproex (Depakote) 250-500 mg PO tid-qid [125, 250, 500 mg].
-Clonazepam (Klonopin) 0.5-5 mg PO bid-qid [0.5, 1, 2 mg].
-Lamotrigine (Lamictal) 50 mg PO qd, then increase to 50-250 mg PO bid [25, 100, 150, 200 mg]; adjunct therapy.

10. **Extras:** MRI with and without gadolinium or CT with contrast; EEG (with photic stimulation, hyperventilation, sleep deprivation, awake and asleep

tracings); portable CXR, ECG.
11. Labs: CBC, SMA 7, glucose, Mg, calcium, phosphate, liver panel, VDRL, anticonvulsant levels. UA, drug screen.

Endocrinologic Disorders

Diabetic Ketoacidosis

1. **Admit to:**
2. **Diagnosis:** Diabetic ketoacidosis
3. **Condition:**
4. **Vital signs:** q1h, postural BP and pulse. Call physician if BP >160/90, <90/60; P >140, <50; R >30, <10; T >38.5°C; or urine output < 20 mL/hr for more than 2 hours.
5. **Activity:** Bed rest with bedside commode.
6. **Nursing:** Inputs and outputs. Foley to closed drainage. Record labs on flow sheet.
7. **Diet:** NPO for 12 hours, then clear liquids as tolerated.
8. **IV Fluids:**

1-2 L NS over 1-3h (≥16 gauge), infuse at 400-1000 mL/h until hemodynamically stable, then change to 0.45% saline at 125-150 cc/hr; keep urine output >30-60 mL/h.

Add KCL when serum potassium is <5.0 mEq/L.

Concentration.......20-40 mEq KCL/L

May use K phosphate, 20-40 mEq/L, in place of KCL if low phosphate.

Change to 5% dextrose in 0.45% saline with 20-40 mEq KCL/liter when blood glucose 250-300.

9. **Special Medications:**
   - -Oxygen at 2 L/min by NC.
   - -Insulin Regular (Humulin) 7-10 units (0.1 U/kg) IV bolus, then 7-10 U/h IV infusion (0.1 U/kg/h); 50 U in 250 mL of 0.9% saline; flush IV tubing with 20 mL of insulin sln before starting infusion. Adjust insulin infusion to decrease serum glucose by 100 mg/dL or less per hour. When bicarbonate level is >16 mEq/L and anion gap <16 mEq/L, decrease insulin infusion rate by half
   - -When the glucose level reaches 250 mg/dL, 5% dextrose should be added to the replacement fluids with KCL 20-40 mEq/L.
   - -Use 10% glucose at 50-100 mL/h if anion gap persists and serum glucose has decreased to less than 100 mg/dL while on insulin infusion.
   - -Change to subcutaneous insulin when anion gap cleared; discontinue insulin infusion 1-2h after subcutaneous dose.
10. **Extras:** Portable CXR, ECG.
11. **Labs:** Fingerstick glucose q1-2h. SMA 7 q4-6h. SMA 12, pH, bicarbonate, phosphate, amylase, lipase, hemoglobin A1c; CBC. UA, serum pregnancy test.

Nonketotic Hyperosmolar Syndrome

1. **Admit to:**
2. **Diagnosis:** Nonketotic hyperosmolar syndrome
3. **Condition:**
4. **Vital signs:** q1h. Call physician if BP >160/90, <90/60; P >140, <50; R>25, <10; T >38.5° C; or urine output <20 cc/hr for more than 4 hours.
5. **Activity:** Bed rest with bedside commode.
6. **Nursing:** Input and output measurement. Foley to closed drainage. Record labs on flow sheet.
7. **Diet:** NPO.
8. **IV Fluids:**
   -1-2 L NS over 1h (≥16 gauge IV catheter), then give 0.45% saline at 125 cc/hr. Maintain urine output ≥50 mL/h.
   -Add 20-40 mEq/L KCL when urine output adequate.
9. **Special Medications:**
   -Insulin regular 2-3 U/h IV infusion (50 U in 250 mL of 0.9% saline).
   -Ranitidine (Zantac) 50 mg IV q8h or 150 mg PO bid.
   -Heparin 5000 U SQ q12h.
10. **Extras:** Portable CXR, ECG.
11. **Labs:** Fingerstick glucose q1-2h x 6h, then q6h. SMA 7, osmolality. SMA 12, phosphate, ketones, hemoglobin A1C, CBC. UA.

Thyroid Storm and Hyperthyroidism

1. **Admit to:**
2. **Diagnosis:** Thyroid Storm
3. **Condition:**
4. **Vital signs:** q1-4h. Call physician if BP >160/90, <90/60; P >130, <50; R>25, <10; T >38.5°C
5. **Activity:** Bed rest
6. **Nursing:** Cooling blanket prn temp >39°C, inputs and outputs. Oxygen 2 L/min by nasal canula.
7. **Diet:** Regular
8. **IV Fluids:** D5 ½ NS at 125 mL/h.
9. **Special Medications:**

Thyroid Storm and Hyperthyroidism:

-Propylthiouracil (PTU) 1000 mg PO, then 50-250 mg PO q4-8h, up to 1200 mg/d; usual maintenance dose 50 mg PO tid **OR**

-Methimazole (Tapazole) 30-60 mg PO, then maintenance of 15 mg PO qd-bid **AND**

-Iodide solution (Lugol's solution), 3-6 drops tid; one hour after propylthiouracil **AND**

-Dexamethasone (Solu-Medrol) 2 mg IV q6h **AND**

-Propranolol 40-160 mg PO q6h or 5-10 mg/h, max 2-5 mg IV q4h or propranolol-LA (Inderal-LA), 80-120 mg PO qd [60, 80, 120, 160 mg].

-Acetaminophen (Tylenol) 1-2 tabs PO q4-6h prn temp >38°C.
-Triazolam (Halcion) 0.125-0.5 mg PO qhs prn sleep **OR**
-Lorazepam (Ativan) 1-2 mg IV/IM/PO q4-8h prn anxiety.

10. Extras: CXR PA and LAT, ECG, endocrine consult. If visual symptoms, obtain ophthalmology consult.

11. Labs: CBC, SMA 7&12; sensitive TSH, free T4. UA.

Myxedema Coma and Hypothyroidism

1. **Admit to:**
2. **Diagnosis:** Myxedema Coma
3. **Condition:**
4. **Vital signs:** q1h. Call physician if BP systolic >160/90, <90/60; P >130, <50; R>25, <10; T >38.5°C
5. **Activity:** Bed rest
6. **Nursing:** Triple blankets prn temp <36°C, inputs and outputs, aspiration precautions.
7. **Diet:** NPO
8. **IV Fluids:** IV D5 NS TKO.
9. **Special Medications:**

Myxedema Coma and Hypothyroidism:

-Volume replacement with NS 1-2 L rapid IV, then 125 mL/h.
-Levothyroxine (Synthroid, Levoxine) 300-500 mcg IV, then 100 mcg PO or IV qd.
-Hydrocortisone 100 mg IV loading dose, then 50-100 mg IV q8h.

Hypothyroidism in Medically Stable Patient:

-Levothyroxine (Synthroid, T4) 50-75 mcg PO qd, increase by 25 mcg PO qd at 2-4 week intervals, to 75-150 mcg qd until TSH normalized.

11. Extras: ECG, endocrine consult.

12. Labs: CBC, SMA 7&12; sensitive TSH, free T4. UA, RA factor, ANA.

Nephrologic Disorders

Renal Failure

1. **Admit to:**
2. **Diagnosis:** Renal Failure
3. **Condition:**
4. **Vital signs:** q8h. Call physician if QRS complex >0.14 sec; urine output <20 cc/hr; BP >160/90, <90/60; P >120, <50; R>25, <10; T >38.5°C
5. **Allergies:** Avoid magnesium containing antacids, salt substitutes, NSAIDS, and other nephrotoxins. Discontinue phosphate or potassium supplements unless depleted.
6. **Activity:** Bed rest.
7. **Nursing:** Daily weights, inputs and outputs, chart urine output. If no urine output for 4h, inputs and outputs catheterize. Guaiac stools.
8. **Diet:** Renal diet of high biologic value protein of 0.6-0.8 g/kg, sodium 2 g, potassium 1 mEq/kg, and at least 35 kcal/kg of nonprotein calories. In oliguric patients, daily fluid intake should be restricted to less than 1 L after volume has been normalized.
9. **IV Fluids:** D5W at TKO.
10. **Special Medications:**
    - -Consider fluid challenge (to rule out pre-renal azotemia if not fluid overloaded) with 500-1000 mL NS IV over 30 min. In acute renal failure, inputs and outputs catheterize and check postvoid residual to rule out obstruction.
    - -Furosemide (Lasix) 80-320 mg IV bolus over 10-60 min, double the dose if no response after 2 hours to total max 1000 mg/24h, or furosemide 1000 mg in 250 mL D5W at 20-40 mg/hr continuous IV infusion **OR**
    - -Torsemide (Demadex) 20-40 mg IV bolus over 5-10 min, double the dose up to max 200 mg/day.
    - -Bumetanide (Bumex) 1-2 mg IV bolus over 1-20 min; double the dose if no response in 1-2 h to total max 10 mg/day.
    - -Metolazone (Zaroxolyn) 5-10 mg PO (max 20 mg/24h) 30 min before a loop diuretic.
    - -Dopamine (Intropin) 1-3 mcg/kg per minute IV.
    - -Hyperkalemia is treated with sodium polystyrene sulfonate (Kayexalate), 15-30 g PO/NG/PR q4-6h.
    - -Hyperphosphatemia is controlled with calcium acetate (Phoslo), 2-3 tabs with meals.
    - -Metabolic acidosis is treated with sodium bicarbonate to maintain the serum pH >7.2 and the bicarbonate level >20 mEq/L. 1-2 amps (50-100 mEq) IV push, followed by infusion of 2-3 amps in 1000 mL of D5W at 150 mL/hr.
    - -Adjust all medications to creatinine clearance, and remove potassium phosphate and magnesium from IV. Avoid NSAIDs and nephrotoxic drugs.
11. **Extras:** CXR, ECG, renal ultrasound, nephrology and dietetics consults.

12. Labs: CBC, platelets, SMA 7&12, creatinine, BUN, potassium, magnesium, phosphate, calcium, uric acid, osmolality, ESR, INR/PTT, ANA.
Urine specific gravity, UA with micro, urine C&S; 1st AM spot urine electrolytes, creatinine, pH, osmolality; Wright's stain, urine electrophoresis. 24h urine protein, creatinine, sodium.

Nephrolithiasis

1. **Admit to:**
2. **Diagnosis:** Nephrolithiasis
3. **Condition:**
4. **Vital signs:** q6h. Call physician if urine output <30 cc/hr; BP >160/90, <90/60; T >38.5°C
5. **Activity:** Up ad lib.
6. **Nursing:** Strain urine, measure inputs and outputs. Place Foley if no urine for 4 hours.
7. **Diet:** Regular, push oral fluids.
8. **IV Fluids:** IV D5 ½ NS at 100-125 cc/hr (maintain urine output of 80 mL/h).
9. **Special Medications:**
   - -Cefazolin (Ancef) 1-2 gm IV q8h
   - -Meperidine (Demerol) 75-100 mg and hydroxyzine 25 mg IM/IV q2-4h prn pain **OR**
   - -Butorphanol (Stadol) 0.5-2 mg IV q3-4h.
   - -Hydrocodone/acetaminophen (Vicodin), 1-2 tab q4-6h PO prn pain **OR**
   - -Hydromorphone (Dilaudid) 1-2 tabs q4-6h PO prn pain **OR**
   - -Acetaminophen with codeine (Tylenol 3) 1-2 tabs PO q3-4h prn pain.
   - -Ketorolac (Toradol) 10 mg PO q4-6h prn pain, or 30-60 mg IV/IM then 15-30 mg IV/IM q6h (max 5 days).
   - -Zolpidem (Ambien) 10 mg PO qhs prn insomnia.

Note: If stone <5 mm without sepsis then discharge home with analgesics and increase PO fluids. If stone >10 mm and/or fever or increased WBC or signs of ureteral dilation, admission for urology evaluation is indicated.

11. Extras: Intravenous pyelogram, KUB, CXR, ECG.

12. Labs: CBC, SMA 6 and 12, calcium, uric acid, phosphorous, UA with micro, urine C&S, urine pH, INR/PTT. Urine cystine (nitroprusside test), send stones for X-ray crystallography. 24 hour urine collection for uric acid, calcium, creatinine.

Hypercalcemia

1. **Admit to:**
2. **Diagnosis:** Hypercalcemia
3. **Condition:**
4. **Vital signs:** q4h. Call physician if BP >160/90, <90/60; P >120, <50; R>25, <10; T >38.5°C; or tetany or any abnormal mental status.
5. **Activity:** Encourage ambulation; up in chair at other times.

6. **Nursing:** Seizure precautions, weigh patient bid, measure inputs and outputs.
7. **Diet:** Restrict dietary calcium to 400 mg/d, push PO fluids.
8. **Special Medications:**
   - -1-2 L of 0.9% saline over 1-4 hours until no longer hypotensive, then saline diuresis with 0.9% saline infused at 125 cc/h **AND**
   - -Furosemide (Lasix) 20-80 mg IV q4-12h. Maintain urine output of 200 mL/h; monitor serum sodium, potassium, magnesium
   - -Calcitonin (Calcimar) 4-8 IV kg IM q12h or SQ q6-12h.
   - -Etidronate (Didronel) 7.5 mg/kg/day in 250 mL of normal saline IV infusion over 2 hours for 3 days.
   - -Pamidronate (Aredia) 60 mg in 1 liter of NS infused over 4 hours or 90 mg in 1 liter of NS infused over 24 hours x one dose.
9. **Extras:** CXR, ECG, mammogram.
10. **Labs:** Total and ionized calcium, SMA 7&12, phosphate, Mg, alkaline phosphatase, prostate specific antigen. 24h urine calcium, phosphate, parathyroid hormone.

Hypocalcemia

1. **Admit to:**
2. **Diagnosis:** Hypocalcemia
3. **Condition:**
4. **Vital signs:** q4h. Call physician if BP >160/90, <90/60; P >120, <50; R>25, <10; T >38.5°C; or any abnormal mental status.
5. **Activity:** Up ad lib
6. **Nursing:** I and O.
7. **Diet:** No added salt diet.
8. **Special Medications:**

Symptomatic Hypocalcemia:
   - -Calcium chloride, 10% (270 mg calcium/10 mL vial) give 5-10 mL slowly over 10 min or dilute in 50-100 mL of D5W and infuse over 20 min, repeat q20-30 min if symptomatic, or hourly if asymptomatic. Correct hyperphosphatemia before hypocalcemia **OR**
   - -Calcium gluconate, 20 mL of 10% solution IV (2 vials)(90 mg elemental calcium/10 mL vial) infused over 10-15 min, followed by infusion of 60 mL of calcium gluconate in 500 cc of D5W (1 mg/mL) at 0.5-2.0 mg/kg/h.

Chronic Hypocalcemia:
   - -Calcium carbonate with vitamin D (Oscal-D) 1-2 tab PO tid **OR**
   - -Calcium carbonate (Oscal) 1-2 tab PO tid **OR**
   - -Calcium citrate (Citracal) 1 tab PO q8h or Extra strength Tums 1-2 PO with meals.
   - -Vitamin D2 (Ergocalciferol) 1 tab PO qd.
   - -Calcitriol (Rocaltrol) 0.25 mcg PO qd, titrate up to 0.5-2.0 mcg qid.
   - -Docusate sodium (Colace) 1 tab PO bid.

9. **Extras:** CXR, ECG.

10. Labs: SMA 7&12, phosphate, Mg. 24h urine calcium, potassium, phosphate, magnesium.

Hyperkalemia

1. **Admit to:**
2. **Diagnosis:** Hyperkalemia
3. **Condition:**
4. **Vital signs:** q4h. Call physician if QRS complex >0.14 sec or BP >160/90, <90/60; P >120, <50; R>25, <10; T >38.5°C.
5. **Activity:** Bed rest; up in chair as tolerated.
6. **Nursing:** Inputs and outputs. Chart QRS complex width q1h.
7. **Diet:** Regular, no salt substitutes.
8. **IV Fluids:** D5NS at 125 cc/h
9. **Special Medications:**
   - -Consider discontinuing ACE inhibitors, angiotensin II receptor blockers, beta-blockers, potassium sparing diuretics.
   - -Calcium gluconate (10% sln) 10-30 mL IV over 2-5 min; second dose may be given in 5 min. Contraindicated if digoxin toxicity is suspected. Keep 10 mL vial of calcium gluconate at bedside for emergent use.
   - -Sodium bicarbonate 1 amp (50 mEq) IV over 5 min (give after calcium in separate IV).
   - -Regular insulin 10 units IV push with 1 ampule of 50% glucose IV push.
   - -Kayexalate 30-45 gm premixed in sorbitol solution PO/NG/PR now and in q3-4h prn, up to 5 times per day.
   - -Furosemide 40-80 mg IV, repeat prn.
   - -Consider emergent dialysis if cardiac complications or renal failure.
10. **Extras:** ECG.
11. **Labs:** CBC, platelets, SMA7, magnesium, calcium, SMA-12. UA, specific gravity, Urine sodium, pH, 24h urine potassium, creatinine.

Hypokalemia

1. **Admit to:**
2. **Diagnosis:** Hypokalemia
3. **Condition:**
4. **Vital signs:** Vitals, urine output q4h. Call physician if BP >160/90, <90/60; P>120, <50; R>25, <10; T >38.5°C.
5. **Activity:** Bed rest; up in chair as tolerated.
6. **Nursing:** Inputs and outputs
7. **Diet:** Regular
8. **Special Medications:**

Acute Therapy:

- -KCL 20-40 mEq in 100 cc saline infused IVPB over 2 hours; or add 40-80 mEq to 1 liter of IV fluid and infuse over 4-8 hours.

-KCL 40 mEq PO tid (in addition to IV); max total dose 100-200 mEq/d (3 mEq/kg/d).

Chronic Therapy:

-KCL elixir 1-3 tablespoon qd-tid PO after meals (20 mEq/Tbsp of 10% sln) **OR**

-Micro-K 10 mEq tabs 2-3 tabs PO tid after meals (40-100 mEq/d) **OR**

-K-Dur 20 mEq tabs 1 PO bid-tid.

Hypokalemia with metabolic acidosis:

-Potassium citrate 15-30 mL in juice PO qid after meals (1 mEq/mL).

-Potassium gluconate 15 mL in juice PO qid after meals (20 mEq/15 mL).

9. Extras: ECG, dietetics consult.

10. Labs: CBC, magnesium, SMA 7&12. UA, urine Na, pH, 24h urine for K, creatinine.

Hypermagnesemia

1. **Admit to:**
2. **Diagnosis:** Hypermagnesemia
3. **Condition:**
4. **Vital signs:** q6h. Call physician if QRS >0.14 sec.
5. **Activity:** Up ad lib
6. **Nursing:** Inputs and outputs, daily weights.
7. **Diet:** Regular
8. **Special Medications:**

   -Saline diuresis 0.9% saline infused at 100-200 cc/h to replace urine loss **AND**

   -Calcium chloride, 1-3 gm added to saline infusate (10% sln; 1 gm per 10 mL amp) to run at 1 gm/hr **AND**

   -Furosemide (Lasix) 20-40 mg IV q4-6h as needed.

   -Magnesium of >9.0 requires stat hemodialysis because of risk of respiratory failure.

9. **Extras:** ECG
10. **Labs:** Magnesium, calcium, SMA 7&12, creatinine. 24 hour urine magnesium, creatinine.

Hypomagnesemia

1. **Admit to:**
2. **Diagnosis:** Hypomagnesemia
3. **Condition:**
4. **Vital signs:** q6h
5. **Activity:** Up ad lib
6. **Diet:** Regular
7. **Special Medications:**

   -Magnesium sulfate 4-6 gm in 500 mL D5W IV at 1 gm/hr. Hold if no patellar reflex. (Estimation of Mg deficit = 0.2 x kg weight x desired increase in Mg concentration; give deficit over 2-3d) **OR**

-Magnesium sulfate (severe hypomagnesemia <1.0) 1-2 gm (2-4 mL of 50% sln) IV over 15 min, **OR**

-Magnesium chloride (Slow-Mag) 65-130 mg (1-2 tabs) PO tid-qid (64 mg or 5.3 mEq/tab) **OR**

-Milk of magnesia 5 mL PO qd-qid.

8. Extras: ECG

9. Labs: Magnesium, calcium, SMA 7&12. Urine Mg, electrolytes, 24h urine magnesium, creatinine.

Hypernatremia

1. **Admit to:**
2. **Diagnosis:** Hypernatremia
3. **Condition:**
4. **Vital signs:** q2h. Call physician if BP >160/90, <70/50; P >140, <50; R>25, <10; T >38.5°C.
5. **Activity:** Bed rest; up in chair as tolerated.
6. **Nursing:** Inputs and outputs, daily weights.
7. **Diet:** No added salt.
8. **Special Medications:**

Hypernatremia with Hypovolemia:

If volume depleted, give 1-2 L NS IV over 1-3 hours until not orthostatic, then give D5W IV or PO to replace half of body water deficit over first 24hours (attempt to correct sodium at 1 mEq/L/h), then remaining deficit over next 1-2 days.

$$\text{Body water deficit (L)} = \frac{0.6(\text{weight kg})([\text{Na serum}]-140)}{140}$$

Hypernatremia with ECF Volume Excess:

-Furosemide 40-80 mg IV or PO qd-bid.

-Salt poor albumin (25%) 50-100 mL bid-tid x 48-72 h.

Hypernatremia with Diabetes Insipidus:

-D5W to correct body water deficit (see above).

-Pitressin 5-10 U IM/IV q6h or desmopressin (DDAVP) 4 mcg IV/SQ q12h; keep urine specific gravity >1.010.

9. Extras: CXR, ECG.

10. Labs: SMA 7&12, serum osmolality, liver panel, ADH, plasma renin activity. UA, urine specific gravity. Urine osmolality, Na, 24h urine K, creatinine.

Hyponatremia

1. **Admit to:**
2. **Diagnosis:** Hyponatremia
3. **Condition:**
4. **Vital signs:** q4h. Call physician if BP >160/90, <70/50; P >140, <50; R>25, <10; T >38.5°C.
5. **Activity:** Up in chair as tolerated.
6. **Nursing:** Inputs and outputs, daily weights.
7. **Diet:** Regular diet.
8. **Special Medications:**

Hyponatremia with Hypervolemia and Edema (low osmolality <280, UNa <10 mmol/L: nephrosis, heart failure, cirrhosis):

-Water restrict to 0.5-1.0 L/d.

-Furosemide 40-80 mg IV or PO qd-bid.

Hyponatremia with Normal Volume Status (low osmolality <280, UNa <10 mmol: water intoxication; UNa >20: SIADH, diuretic-induced):

-Water restrict to 0.5-1.5 L/d.

Hyponatremia with Hypovolemia (low osmolality <280) UNa <10 mmol/L: vomiting, diarrhea, third space/respiratory/skin loss; UNa >20 mmol/L: diuretics, renal injury, RTA, adrenal insufficiency, partial obstruction, salt wasting:

- If volume depleted, give 0.5-2 L of 0.9% saline over 1-2 hours until no longer hypotensive, then 0.9% saline at 125 cc/h or 100-500 cc 3% hypertonic saline over 4h.

Severe Symptomatic Hyponatremia:

If volume depleted, give 1-2 L of 0.9% saline (154 mEq/L) over 1-2 hours until no longer orthostatic.

Determine volume of 3% hypertonic saline (513 mEq/L) to be infused:

Na (mEq) deficit = 0.6 x (wt kg)x(desired [Na] - actual [Na])

$$\frac{\text{Volume of sln (L)}}{\text{Number of hrs}} = \frac{\text{Sodium to be infused (mEq)}}{\text{(mEq/L in sln) x Number of hrs}}$$

-Correct half of sodium deficit intravenously over 24 hours until serum sodium is 120 mEq/L; increase sodium by 12-20 mEq/L over 24 hours (1 mEq/L/h).

-Alternative Method: 3% saline 100-300 cc over 4-6h, repeated as needed.

9. **Extras:** CXR, ECG, head/chest CT scan.
10. **Labs:** SMA 7&12, osmolality, triglyceride, liver panel. UA, urine specific gravity. Urine osmolality, Na.

Hyperphosphatemia

1. **Admit to:**
2. **Diagnosis:** Hyperphosphatemia
3. **Condition:**
4. **Vital signs:** qid
5. **Activity:** Up ad lib
6. **Nursing:** Inputs and outputs
7. **Diet:** Low phosphorus diet with 0.7-1 gm/d
8. **Special Medications:**

Moderate Hyperphosphatemia:

-Restrict dietary phosphate to 0.7-1.0 gm/d.
-Calcium acetate (Phoslo) 1-3 tabs PO tid with meals, **OR**
-Aluminum hydroxide (Amphojel) 5-10 mL or 1-2 tablets PO before meals tid.

Severe Hyperphosphatemia:

-Volume expansion with 0.9% saline 1-2 L over 1-2h.
-Acetazolamide (Diamox) 500 mg PO or IV q6h.
-Consider dialysis.

9. **Extras:** CXR PA and LAT, ECG.
10. **Labs:** Phosphate, SMA 7&12, magnesium, calcium. UA, parathyroid hormone.

Hypophosphatemia

1. **Admit to:**
2. **Diagnosis:** Hypophosphatemia
3. **Condition:**
4. **Vital signs:** qid
5. **Activity:** Up ad lib
6. **Nursing:** Inputs and outputs.
7. **Diet:** Regular diet.
8. **Special Medications:**

Mild to Moderate Hypophosphatemia (1.0-2.2 mg/dL):

-Sodium or potassium phosphate 0.25 mMoles/kg in 150-250 mL of NS or D5W at 10 mMoles/h.
-Neutral phosphate (Nutra-Phos), 2 tab PO bid (250 mg elemental phosphorus/tab) **OR**
-Phospho-Soda 5 mL (129 mg phosphorus) PO bid-tid.

Severe Hypophosphatemia (<1.0 mg/dL):

-Na or K phosphate 0.5 mMoles/kg in 250 mL D5W or NS, IV infusion at 10 mMoles/hr **OR**
-Add potassium phosphate to IV solution in place of maintenance KCL; max IV dose 7.5 mg phosphorus/kg/6h.

9. **Extras:** CXR PA and LAT, ECG.
10. **Labs:** Phosphate, SMA 7&12, Mg, calcium, UA.

Rheumatologic Disorders

Systemic Lupus Erythematosus

1. **Admit to:**
2. **Diagnosis:** Systemic Lupus Erythematosus
3. **Condition:**
4. **Vital signs:** tid
5. **Allergies:**
6. **Activity:** Up as tolerated with bathroom privileges
7. **Nursing:**
8. **Diet:** No added salt, low psoralen diet.
9. **Special Medications:**
   -Ibuprofen (Motrin) 400 mg PO qid (max 2.4 g/d) **OR**
   -Indomethacin (Indocin) 25-50 mg tid-qid.
   -Hydroxychloroquine (Plaquenil) 200-600 mg/d PO
   -Prednisone 60-100 mg PO qd, may increase to 200-300 mg/d. Maintenance 10-20 mg PO qd or 20-40 mg PO qOD **OR**
   -Methylprednisolone (pulse therapy) 500 mg IV over 30 min q12h for 3-5d, then prednisone 50 mg PO qd.
   -Betamethasone dipropionate (Diprolene) 0.05% ointment applied bid.
10. **Extras:** CXR PA, LAT, ECG. Rheumatology consult.
11. **Labs:** CBC, platelets, SMA 7&12, INR/PTT, ESR, complement CH-50, C3, C4, C-reactive protein, LE prep, Coombs test, VDRL, rheumatoid factor, ANA, DNA binding, lupus anticoagulant, anticardiolipin, antinuclear cytoplasmic antibody. UA.

Acute Gout Attack

1. **Admit to:**
2. **Diagnosis:** Acute gout attack
3. **Condition:**
4. **Vital signs:** tid
5. **Activity:** Bed rest with bedside commode
6. **Nursing:** Keep foot elevated; support sheets over foot; guaiac stools.
7. **Diet:** Low purine diet.
8. **Special Medications:**
   -Ibuprofen (Motrin) 800 mg, then 400-800 mg PO q4-6h **OR**
   -Diclofenac (Voltaren) 25-75 mg tid-qid with food **OR**
   -Indomethacin (Indocin) 25-50 mg PO q6h for 2d, then 50 mg tid for 2 days, then 25 mg PO tid **OR**
   -Ketorolac (Toradol) 30-60 mg IV/IM, then 15-30 mg IV/IM q6h or 10 mg PO tid-qid **OR**

-Naproxen sodium (Anaprox, Anaprox-DS) 550 mg PO bid **OR**
-Methylprednisolone (SoluMedrol) 125 mg IV x 1 dose **THEN**
-Prednisone 60 mg PO qd for 5 days, followed by tapering.
-Colchicine 2 tablets (0.5 mg or 0.6 mg), followed by 1 tablet q1h until relief, max dose of 9.6 mg/24h. Maintenance colchicine: 0.5-0.6 mg PO qd-bid.

Hypouricemic Therapy:

-Probenecid (Benemid), 250 mg bid. Increase the dosage to 500 mg bid after 1 week, then increase by 500-mg increments every 4 weeks until the uric acid level is below 6.5 mg/dL. Max dose 2 g/d. Contraindicated during acute attack.
-Allopurinol (Zyloprim) 300 mg PO qd, may increase by 100-300 mg q2weeks. Usually initiated after the acute attack.

9. Symptomatic Medications:

-Ranitidine (Zantac) 150 mg PO bid.
-Meperidine (Demerol) 50-100 mg IM/IV q4-6h prn pain **OR**
-Hydrocodone/acetaminophen (Vicodin), 1-2 tab q4-6h PO prn pain

10. Labs: CBC, SMA 7, uric acid. UA with micro. Synovial fluid for light and polarizing micrography for crystals; C&S, Gram stain, glucose, protein, cell count. X-ray views of joint. 24 hour urine for uric acid.

Commonly Used Formulas

A-a gradient = $[(P_B\text{-}PH_2O)\ FiO_2 - PCO_2/R] - PO_2$ arterial

$= (713 \times FiO_2 - pCO_2/0.8) - pO_2$ arterial

$P_B = 760$ mmHg; $PH_2O = 47$ mmHg ; $R = 0.8$
normal Aa gradient <10-15 mmHg (room air)

Arterial oxygen capacity =(Hgb(gm)/100 mL) x 1.36 mL O_2/gm Hgb

Arterial O_2 content = $1.36(Hgb)(SaO_2)+0.003(PaO_2)$= NL 20 vol%

O_2 delivery = CO x arterial O_2 content = NL 640-1000 mL O_2/min

Cardiac output = HR x stroke volume

$$\text{CO L/min} = \frac{125 \text{ mL } O_2/\text{min}/M^2}{8.5\ \{(1.36)(Hgb)(SaO_2) - (1.36)(Hgb)(SvO_2)\}} \times 100$$

Normal CO = 4-6 L/min

Na (mEq) deficit = 0.6 x (wt kg) x (desired [Na] - actual [Na])

$$\text{SVR} = \frac{\text{MAP - CVP}}{CO_{L/min}} \times 80 = \text{NL 800-1200 dyne/sec/cm}^2$$

$$\text{PVR} = \frac{\text{PA - PCWP}}{CO_{L/min}} \times 80 = \text{NL 45-120 dyne/sec/cm}^2$$

$$\text{GFR mL/min} = \frac{(140 - \text{age}) \times \text{ideal weight in kg}}{72 \text{ (males)} \times \text{serum creatinine (mg/dL)}}$$
85 (females) x serum creatinine (mg/dL)

$$\text{Creatinine clearance} = \frac{\text{U creatinine (mg/100 mL)} \times \text{U vol (mL)}}{\text{P creatinine (mg/100 mL)} \times \text{time (1440 min for 24h)}}$$

Normal creatinine clearance = 100-125 mL/min(males), 85-105(females)

$$\text{Body water deficit (L)} = \frac{0.6(\text{weight kg})([\text{measured serum Na}]-140)}{140}$$

$$\text{Serum Osmolality} = 2\,[Na] + \frac{BUN}{2.8} + \frac{Glucose}{18} = 270\text{-}290$$

Na (mEq) deficit = 0.6 x (wt kg)x(desired [Na] - actual [Na])

$$\text{Fractional excreted Na} = \frac{\text{U Na/ Serum Na} \times 100}{\text{U creatinine/ Serum creatinine}} = \text{NL}<1\%$$

Anion Gap = Na - ($Cl + HCO_3$)

For each 100 mg/dL increase in glucose, Na decreases by 1.6 mEq/L.

Corrected serum Ca^+ (mg/dL) = measured Ca mg/dL + 0.8 x (4 - albumin g/dL)

Predicted Maximal Heart Rate = 220 - age

Normal ECG Intervals (sec)

PR	0.12-0.20
QRS	0.06-0.08
Heart rate/min	**Q-T**
60	0.33-0.43
70	0.31-0.41
80	0.29-0.38
90	0.28-0.36
100	0.27-0.35

Total Parenteral Nutrition Equations:

Caloric Requirements: (Harris-Benedict Equations)

Basal energy expenditure (BEE)

Females: 655 + (9.6 x wt in kg) + (1.85 x ht in cm) - (4.7 x age)

Males: 66 + (13.7 x wt in kg) + (5 x ht in cm) - (6.8 x age)

A. BEE x 1.2 = Caloric requirement for minimally stressed patient
B. BEE x 1.3 = Caloric requirement for moderately stressed patient (inflammatory bowel disease, cancer, surgery)
C. BEE x 1.5 = Caloric requirement for severely stressed patient (major sepsis, burns, AIDS, liver disease)
D. BEE x 1.7 = Caloric requirement for extremely stressed patient (traumatic burns >50%, open head trauma, multiple stress)

Protein Requirements:

A. Protein requirement for non-stressed patient = 0.8 gm protein/kg.
B. Protein requirement for patients with decreased visceral protein states (hypoalbuminemia), recent weight loss, or hypercatabolic states = 1.0-1.5 gm protein/kg.

Estimation of Ideal Body Weight:

A. Females: 5 feet (allow 100 lbs) + 5 lbs for each inch over 5 feet
B. Males: 5 feet (allow 106 lbs) + 6 lbs for each inch over 5 feet

Commonly Used Drug Levels

Drug	Therapeutic Range
Amikacin	Peak 25-30; trough <10 mcg/mL
Amiodarone	1.0-3.0 mcg/mL
Amitriptyline	100-250 ng/mL
Carbamazepine	4-10 mcg/mL
Desipramine	150-300 ng/mL
Digoxin	0.8-2.0 ng/mL
Disopyramide	2-5 mcg/mL
Doxepin	75-200 ng/mL
Flecainide	0.2-1.0 mcg/mL
Gentamicin	Peak 6.0-8.0; trough <2.0 mcg/mL
Imipramine	150-300 ng/mL
Lidocaine	2-5 mcg/mL
Lithium	0.5-1.4 mEq/L
Mexiletine	1.0-2.0 mcg/mL
Nortriptyline	50-150 ng/mL
Phenobarbital	10-30 mEq/mL
Phenytoin	8-20 mcg/mL
Procainamide	4.0-8.0 mcg/mL
Quinidine	2.5-5.0 mcg/mL
Salicylate	15-25 mg/dL
Streptomycin	Peak 10-20; trough <5 mcg/mL
Theophylline	8-20 mcg/mL
Tocainide	4-10 mcg/mL
Valproic acid	50-100 mcg/mL
Vancomycin	Peak 30-40; trough <10 mcg/mL

Extended Interval Gentamicin and Tobramycin Dosing

Estimate the glomerular filtration rate as follows:

Estimated GFR (mL/min) for males $= \dfrac{(140 - \text{age}) \times \text{ideal weight in kg}}{72 \times \text{serum creatinine (mg/dL)}}$

Estimated GFR (mL/min) for females $= \dfrac{(140 - \text{age}) \times \text{ideal weight in kg}}{85 \times \text{serum creatinine (mg/dL)}}$

Extended Interval Gentamicin/Tobramycin Therapy

GFR (mL/min)	Gentamicin/Tobramycin Dosage Frequency
>60	7 mg/kg every 24 hours
40-59	7 mg/kg every 36 hours
20-39	7 mg/kg every 48 hours
<20	Extended interval not recommended
Each dose is administer over 60 minutes. Therapeutic range is a peak level of 20-30 mcg/mL and a trough level of <1.0 mcg/mL (during the 4 hours before the next dose). Monitor renal function and hearing status.	

Commonly Used Abbreviations

1/2 NS — 0.45% saline solution
ac — ante cibum (before meals)
ABG — arterial blood gas
ac — before meals
ACTH — adrenocorticotropic hormone
ad lib — ad libitum (as needed or desired)
ADH — antidiuretic hormone
AFB — acid-fast bacillus
alk phos — alkaline phosphatase
ALT — alanine aminotransferase
am — morning
AMA — against medical advice
amp — ampule
AMV — assisted mandatory ventilation; assist mode ventilation
ANA — antinuclear antibody
ante — before
AP — anteroposterior
ARDS — adult respiratory distress syndrome
ASA — acetylsalicylic acid
AST — aspartate aminotransferase
bid — bis in die (twice a day)
B-12 — vitamin B-12 (cyanocobalamin)
BM — bowel movement
BP — blood pressure
BUN — blood urea nitrogen
c/o — complaint of
c — cum (with)
C and S — culture and sensitivity
C — centigrade
Ca — calcium
cap — capsule
CBC — complete blood count; includes hemoglobin, hematocrit, red blood cell indices, white blood cell count, and platelets
cc — cubic centimeter
CCU — coronary care unit
cm — centimeter
CMF — cyclophosphamide, methotrexate, fluorouracil
CNS — central nervous system
CO_2 — carbon dioxide
COPD — chronic obstructive pulmonary disease
CPK-MB — myocardial-specific CPK isoenzyme
CPR — cardiopulmonary resuscitation
CSF — cerebrospinal fluid
CT — computerized tomography
CVP — central venous pressure
CXR — chest x-ray
d/c — discharge; discontinue
D5W — 5% dextrose water solution; also D10W, D50W
DIC — disseminated intravascular coagulation
diff — differential count
DKA — diabetic ketoacidosis
dL — deciliter
DOSS — docusate sodium sulfosuccinate
DT's — delirium tremens
ECG — electrocardiogram
ER — emergency room
ERCP — endoscopic retrograde cholangiopancreatography
ESR — erythrocyte sedimentation rate
ET — endotracheal tube
ETOH — alcohol
FEV_1 — forced expiratory volume (in one second)
FiO2 — fractional inspired oxygen
g — gram(s)
GC — gonococcal; gonococcus
GFR — glomerular filtration rate
GI — gastrointestinal
gm — gram
gt — drop
gtt — drops
h — hour
H20 — water
HBsAG — hepatitis B surface antigen
HCO3 — bicarbonate
Hct — hematocrit
HDL — high-density lipoprotein
Hg — mercury
Hgb — hemoglobin concentration
HIV — human immunodeficiency virus
hr — hour
hs — hora somni (bedtime, hour of sleep)
IM — intramuscular
I and O — intake and output--measurement of the patient's intake and output, including urine, vomit, diarrhea, and drainage

IU	international units
ICU	intensive care unit
IgM	immunoglobulin M
IMV	intermittent mandatory ventilation
INH	isoniazid
INR	International normalized ratio
IPPB	intermittent positive-pressure breathing
IV	intravenous or intravenously
IVP	intravenous pyelogram; intravenous piggyback
K^+	potassium
kcal	kilocalorie
KCL	potassium chloride
KPO4	potassium phosphate
KUB	x-ray of abdomen (kidneys, ureters, bowels)
L	liter
LDH	lactate dehydrogenase
LDL	low-density lipoprotein
liq	liquid
LLQ	left lower quadrant
LP	lumbar puncture, low potency
LR	lactated Ringer's (solution)
MB	myocardial band
MBC	minimal bacterial concentration
mcg	microgram
mEq	milliequivalent
mg	milligram
Mg	magnesium
MgSO4	Magnesium Sulfate
MI	myocardial infarction
MIC	minimum inhibitory concentration
mL	milliliter
mm	millimeter
MOM	Milk of Magnesia
MRI	magnetic resonance imaging
Na	sodium
NaHCO3	sodium bicarbonate
Neuro	neurologic
NG	nasogastric
NKA	no known allergies
NPH	neutral protamine Hagedorn (insulin)
NPO	nulla per os (nothing by mouth)
NS	normal saline solution (0.9%)
NSAID	nonsteroidal anti-inflammatory drug
O2	oxygen
OD	right eye
oint	ointment
OS	left eye
Osm	osmolality
OT	occupational therapy
OTC	over the counter
OU	each eye
oz	ounce
p, post	after
pc	post cibum (after meals)
PA	posteroanterior; pulmonary artery
PaO2	arterial oxygen pressure
pAO2	partial pressure of oxygen in alveolar gas
PB	phenobarbital
pc	after meals
pCO2	partial pressure of carbon dioxide
PEEP	positive end-expiratory pressure
per	by
pH	hydrogen ion concentration (H+)
PID	pelvic inflammatory disease
pm	afternoon
PO	orally, per os
pO2	partial pressure of oxygen
polys	polymorphonuclear leukocytes
PPD	purified protein derivative
PR	per rectum
prn	pro re nata (as needed)
PT	physical therapy; prothrombin time
PTCA	percutaneous transluminal coronary angioplasty
PTT	partial thromboplastin time
PVC	premature ventricular contraction
q	quaque (every) q6h, q2h every 6 hours; every 2 hours
qid	quarter in die (four times a day)
qAM	every morning
qd	quaque die (every day)
qh	every hour
qhs	every night before bedtime
qid	4 times a day
qOD	every other day
qs	quantity sufficient
R/O	rule out
RA	rheumatoid arthritis; room air; right atrial
Resp	respiratory rate
RL	Ringer's lactated solution (also LR)
ROM	range of motion

rt	right
s	sine (without)
s/p	status post (the condition of being after)
sat	saturated
SBP	systolic blood pressure
SC	subcutaneously
SIADH	syndrome of inappropriate antidiuretic hormone
SL	sublingually under tongue
SLE	systemic lupus erythematosus
SMA-12	sequential multiple analysis; a panel of 12 chemistry tests. Tests include Na^+, K^+, HCO3 , chloride, BUN, glucose, creatinine, bilirubin, calcium, total protein, albumin, and alkaline phosphatase. Other chemistry panels include SMA-6 and SMA-20
SMX	sulfamethoxazole
sob	shortness of breath
sol	solution
SQ	under the skin
ss	one-half
STAT	statim (immediately)
susp	suspension
tid	ter in die (three times a day)
T4	Thyroxine level (T4)
T3RU	Triiodothyronine resin uptake
tab	tablet
TB	tuberculosis
Tbsp	tablespoon
Temp	temperature
TIA	transient ischemic attack
tid	three times a day
TKO	to keep open, an infusion rate (500 mL/24h) just enough to keep the IV from clotting
TMP	trimethoprim
TMP-SMX	trimethoprim-sulfamethoxazole combination
TPA	tissue plasminogen activator
TSH	thyroid-stimulating hormone
tsp	teaspoon
U	units
UA	urinalysis
ung	ointment
URI	upper respiratory infection
Ut Dict	as directed
UTI	urinary tract infection
VAC	vincristine, adriamycin, and cyclophosphamide
vag	vaginal
VC	vital capacity
VDRL	Venereal Disease Research Laboratory
VF	ventricular function
V fib	ventricular fibrillation
VLDL	very low-density lipoprotein
Vol	volume
VS	vital signs
VT	ventricular tachycardia
W	water
WBC	white blood count
x	times

Index

Internet Journals from
Current Clinical Strategies Publishing

Journal of Primary Care Medicine
Journal of Medicine
Journal of Pediatrics and Adolescent Medicine
Journal of Surgery
Journal of Family Medicine
Journal of Emergency Medicine and Acute Primary Care
Journal of Psychiatry
Journal of AIDS/HIV

---

www.ccspublishing.com